Praise
Food

MW00978011

Jill has massively changed the way I view weight, food, and my body. She taught me to trust my intuition and the signals my body gives me. Many times what I'm craving is not food, it's something else. When I go find that something else, love, connection, play, I give my whole self what it needs, not the hollow substitute of food. The freedom that has come from changing my frame of reference is incredible. I'm so excited Jill is sharing these concepts on a wider stage and that other women and men will be able to take the same journey.

— Emily Chase Smith, Esq,
CEO, Chase Smith Press, Inc.
ChaseSmithPress.com

Food for the Journey is a brilliant and practical blend of weight loss science and mindset, making it an essential companion to any weight loss plan. Jill gives you step-by-step instructions for choosing a plan that will work for your unique history, personality, and daily tendencies to help you become the healthiest version of you.

— Nick Pavlidis
Vice President / Chief Terrible Husband
Author of Confessions of a Terrible Husband

Jill is a master at helping people change their perspective on their inner core well being. I love how she teaches people to love "their soul style." Her enthusiasm to see women grow into a stronger version of themselves is really inspiring.

— Jen McDonough (aka The Iron Jen)
Amazon Top 100 Author, Motivational Storyteller
TheIronJen.com

Through Jill's own struggles she has learned it's not about the food, it's not about diets, it's not about anyone else; it's about LOVE. Self love. Nourishing yourself—body, mind, and soul. And she can teach you to do the same.

— Diana Bader
Fresh Canvas, LLC
FreshCanvasCoaching.com

Brave, Beautiful You. That phrase completely captures who Jill Davis is and what she helps her coaching clients become.

— Kent Julian
Founder, LiveItForward.com

Jill Davis taught me that selfish isn't a bad word. She taught me that failure is an opportunity to learn more about myself and understand myself. Jill's coaching changed my life. I went from virtually no relationships to abundant love, forgiveness, and a life full of love and people, on my terms... and she gave me the gift of soul sisterhood.

— Jessica Arent
Soul Sister

Jill was the first woman in my life who taught me how to value myself. She asked me the all-important question, "Do you have a deserve level?" At the time, I didn't even understand the question. But it began my journey of becoming an emotionally healthy human being. It was in part due to her love and support of who I was and could be—at my most broken stage—that allowed me to become all that I am. I live life now with confidence and knowing I have choices. I now understand and love the woman of strength I was created to be.

— Katie Pierce
Client

Jill's open heart and her generosity in reaching out to me just when my life needed it most was wonderfully refreshing. She is the real deal and her story inspires and motivates those who need her message the most. It was no accident we met. It was a blessing.

— Laurie Wilson
Client
Partner, Steve Weed Fine Art, Colorado Springs
SteveWeed.com

Jill Davis has perfected the art of serving the world with her professional skills while adding the personal touch of a dear friend. She wears her passion for women's issues and her love for those she serves as a beacon of hope for all who dare to discover their best self. I am honored to call her a mentor and friend.

— Beth Underwood
Award-Winning Author and Historical Writer
BethWrightUnderwood.com

Jill is gracious in truth telling and she understands where we have come from because she has been there. She is compassionate, thoughtful, experienced, and knowledgeable, while challenging you to be the best you can be!

— Robin Stephenson, M.Ed
CEO, V-Suites Colorado Springs
v-suitescs.com

Jill's philosophy about food and health comes from her personal experience. She has lived her book. I remember asking Jill how she had lost so much weight. "I stopped eating my anger." That line reminds me more than 10 years later not to feed emotion. She also taught me that food did not have morality. Food is morally neutral. I am not of good or bad moral character based on the foods I eat. I appreciate her authenticity as it creates trust for those who work with her and who will read this book.

— Christine Fletcher
REALTOR®
Christine4Houses.com

Jill Davis is a breath of fresh air! Her program is a refreshing change from the self-hating cycle of dieting. Not only do you lose weight and feel healthier, you fall in love with who you are on the inside!

— Heather Woosley
Mom, Fiber Art Instructor, and Musician

Jill is an inspiration! Her heartfelt honesty in sharing her life journey has helped many people as they have watched her make lemonade out of lemons! Jill teaches how to lead an authentic life by being true to yourself! You will be blessed by every word in this book!

— Shari Guest
Client

To be able to get to the bottom of the issue a person is struggling with is a gift. Jill has that gift. Her insight, advice, council, and leadership are delivered so gently and lovingly and always right on target. Her coaching is filled with encouragement, truth, and persistence.

— Carolyn Selvig
Client

I spent most of my life in trauma and developed a lot of bad habits as an escape. When I gave up the alcohol and cigarettes I used food to avoid the feelings of craziness. I wanted no part of feeling my "feelings" because it made me feel out of control. I started coaching with Jill and she was the first person to ask me, "How does that make you feel?"

I still don't like to think about that "touchy-feely crap." Jill helped me realize that there is value in our feelings; that it's important to listen to our feelings and our bodies as they were both given to us as a gift for very specific purposes. This book is as close to coaching with Jill as possible. She puts her thoughts and heart together in an easily to follow process.

— Rhonda Koehn
Client, Hairstylist/ Cosmetology Instructor
Enid Beauty College

Food for the Journey
Stop Fighting Your Weight
Start Finding Your Way

Jill Davis
JillDavisCoaching.com

FREE AGENT PRESS
SATSUMA, ALABAMA

Food for the Journey:
Stop Fighting Your Weight, Start Finding Your Way

© 2016 by Jill Davis, JillDavisCoaching.com
Published by Free Agent Press, FreeAgentPress.com
Satsuma, Alabama 36572
VID: 20161024

While the author has made every effort to provide accurate Internet addresses throughout the text, neither the publisher nor the author assumes any responsibility for errors, or for changes that occur after publication. Further, the author and publisher do not have any control over and do not assume any responsibility for third-party websites or their content.

ISBN-13: 978-0-9982746-0-7
ISBN-10: 0-9982746-0-7

Edited by Jennifer Harshman, HarshmanServices.com
Cover Photo by Megan Miks, MeganMiksPhotography.com
Layout & Cover Design by James Woosley, FreeAgentPress.com
Back Cover & Author Photo by Kerry Kruegler, KerryKruegler.com

To my four beautiful children:
Mark Packard
David Packard
Jacob Packard
Gracie Packard

Because of you I learned unconditional love;
how to give it and how to receive it.

You are my heart.

CONTENTS

It's easier to be brave when
a friend is holding your hand.
— Jill Davis

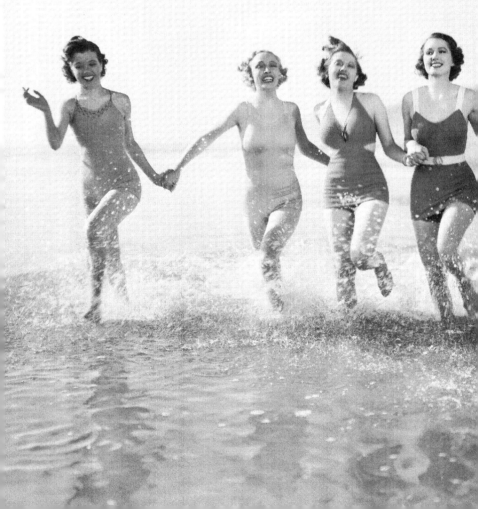

Dear Brave, Beautiful You:

WELCOME TO THIS journey on the way to **your** natural and healthy weight. I am so glad you have chosen to see what's here. It may be that you purchased this title because you really want to love yourself, you are ready for change, you are intrigued by the concept of true weight loss, someone told you that you need to lose weight, or perhaps you just really hope this time you can *finally* be done with thinking about food all the time. Whatever your reason, I am glad you have joined me.

Although many people call this process weight loss, I prefer weight release. This is simply because when I lose something, I always want to find it again. I lose my keys and other assorted items on a regular basis. My hope is that they will show up again and show up again soon. When I lost weight in the past, that is exactly what happened: the weight showed up again and again and again. This time I've kept off 130 pounds for almost ten years.

I have been on so many diets in my lifetime. I have dieted over and over and over again. Until the day came when I decided no more dieting. That day happened in 2006. It's been a journey since then. Through that journey, I was able to fit back into my size 18 skinny jeans from my younger years. Then I went all the way back to a size 10, then even lower. And sometimes I went back up. Through my journey, I learned much about my body and myself.

The journey took me to a place where I learned to connect my soul, mind, and body. I gave up being too aware of my jeans size and learned to embrace the size of my soul. I learned how to eat M&M's and keep the weight off, but more importantly I learned to embrace my body and love my body all of the time. I also learned to like my body at least most of the time.

My hope is that by putting all of this into words, you will be able to shorten your learning curve. You will be able to move into your soul size and truly fall in love with your body and your life as you meld your body, mind, and soul, and become the brave, beautiful self that you are.

With so much love and gratitude for you and your journey,

ENJOY TODAY!
There will never be
another like it.
— Jill Davis

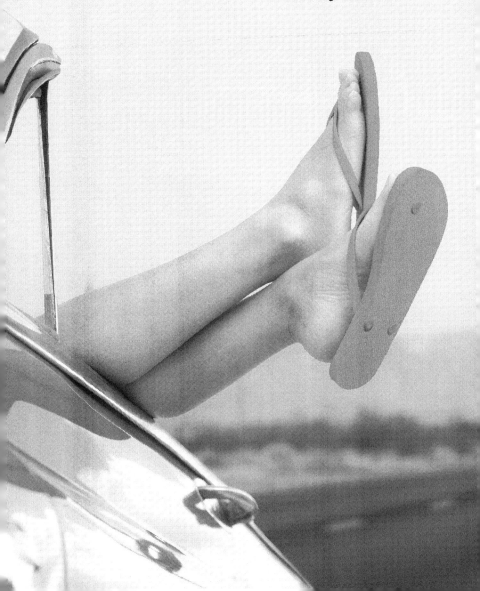

MEDICAL DISCLAIMER

Y EP, I HAVE to do that legal thing. Thanks for reading this piece.

This book provides weight-loss information and is only intended to assist readers in their personal weight-loss efforts. Nothing contained in this book is medical advice or diagnosis nor should any information on my website be construed as such. While my weight loss is the actual result of falling in love with my life, results are not guaranteed.

Individual weight-loss results, amount, and time duration will vary.

You are urged and advised to seek the advice of a physician before beginning any weight-loss effort or program. The advice in this book is not intended for use by minors, pregnant women, or individuals with certain health conditions. Such individuals are specifically warned to seek professional medical advice prior to initiating any type of weight-loss effort.

Weight loss can create physical changes that should be professionally monitored. Medical monitoring is especially important for people with a known medical condition. If you are currently being treated for an illness, taking any prescription medications, following a specialized diet plan to treat a disease, or living with a known medical condition, it's especially important to talk to your physician before attempting any weight-loss program. Any plan modifications by your physician should be followed.

YAY!!! YOU'RE HERE!!!
Let's go!
YOU ARE COURAGEOUS!!!

I am so glad we share the same world!
Brave, Beautiful, YOU!
I am grateful!
—Jill Davis

JILL'S DISCLAIMER

I HAVE A ZERO-TOLERANCE policy for bullying. Most of us spend our lives saying things to the reflection of our inner selves that we would NEVER say to others. Some of my favorites are:

- "How did you get so fat?"
- "What's wrong with you, you lazy bum?"
- "You're never going to look good."
- "Why do you even bother?"

Even as you read this book, you will most likely feel some of these emotions and hear your own specific brand of hurting words. Even now after 130 pounds of weight release, I can occasionally fall back into the habit of being mean to myself. When being mean to ourselves—bullying—becomes a habit, we feel the pain but are no longer conscious of the cause. It's time to become conscious of kindness to yourself.

My zero-tolerance policy doesn't mean you will get struck by lightning if you are mean to yourself, nor will I track you down to scold you. It just means that if you fall into that habit, it will be greeted with love, grace, and acceptance, but know that I won't be agreeing with you.

You are important to me and I won't you let talk badly about my friend. I hope you can offer the same to yourself. You are important in this world. You are beautifully brave.

Fall in love
with your life.
It changes
everything.
— Jill Davis

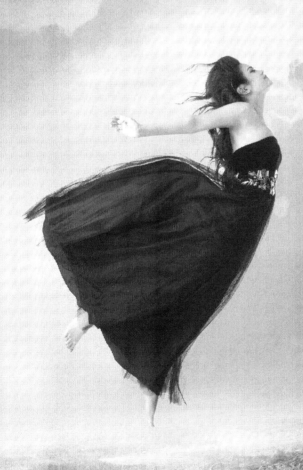

CHAPTER 1

To live will be an awfully big adventure.

— J. M. Barrie

OUR ADVENTURE IN LIFE—OUR story—begins long before we are able to consciously decide what we will choose to take with us and what we will choose to release. Our childhoods are the beginning of the definition of who we are and who we are going to be. Our family position also has much to do with how we perceive life. I am the youngest of six siblings in a family that also included many foster children. This is how my adventure began.

Of my mother's six biological children, I was the only one who resembled my father's side of the family. My father's side was the "heavy" side. His sister was both beautiful as well as morbidly obese. During my childhood, everyone commented on how much I looked just like her and in truth, we did have many features in common. However, as a child, I was unable to connect to her beauty, but I connected to her weight. As long as I can remember, I felt a little bigger than everyone else, even though I wasn't. The thought that I was fat was deeply imprinted in my soul.

I grew up in the foothills of Colorado. Playing on the prairies, swimming in the creeks, climbing trees, exploring the mountains, and loving the beauty of nature; this is the adventure that was my childhood.

Somehow I went from being that adventurous little girl to a teenager who constantly worried about her weight to a woman who weighed over 255 pounds.

Around fifth grade, I did this crazy thing and I got really, really big and tall. I went from five feet tall to five foot four in three months! I went from 85 pounds to 105 pounds in four months. Although I wasn't really that big, it happened so fast my mom began to worry about me. I was definitely taller and bigger than my five foot three mom and my sisters who were both shorter than she.

My beautiful mother, who loved me so much, was a true '60s/'70s mom. She was born in 1925 and she grew up with the concept that thin women are happier, and more importantly, thin women get married more easily. So when she saw her precious little girl get so big so fast, she put me on a diet. I became one of those weight-watching kids and was put on a highly restrictive diet. I didn't know until years later how restrictive it was. I got to eat four to five diet bars a day and drink two diet sodas. It equaled out to about 880 calories.

We know *now* that 880 calories a day is not enough to subsist on. It's certainly not enough for a growing little girl—who loved to run and play and dance—to live on. It's not really enough for anyone to live on. But in 1972, that was not common knowledge. My mother had no idea that she was being too restrictive. She simply loved me very much and wanted the best for me.

At the time, our small elementary school had a wonderful cook that prepared all the students' lunches in the school kitchen. It was not the mass food that is now served in schools. Not only was the food delicious, it was also nutritious and well balanced. I could smell and see the wonderful food, but because skinniness was so important in my world, I began to starve myself. I was a "good girl" who followed the rules; it never occurred to me to ignore my mom's wishes and eat extra food at school.

I had entered the world of women participating in the great famine of dieting. I maintained my weight of about 105 pounds through tenth grade by fighting the desire to eat and by working out a lot. The summer between ninth and tenth grades was a difficult one. I experienced many personal and family transitions.

For the first time ever, there were not siblings everywhere. My sister (who was four years older) had headed off to college and independent living. My other sister (who was just two years older) was on a foreign-student exchange program. Because this was the first time I had been an only child, I spent lots of time on my own and learned to mask the pain I felt with food and sugar.

I had become used to the kinds of chaos that happens when there are many children in a family. When my sisters left home, that chaos reduced and my need for the adrenaline rush that came with it was replaced with food.

We now know that white sugar and simple carbohydrates can help increase certain neurotransmitters in our brains and temporarily make us feel better.[1] I didn't know the chemistry behind it; I just knew I felt better when I was eating peanut M&M's and drinking Diet Coke.

Over that summer I "ballooned" up to 140 pounds. My mother offered me a $200 shopping spree to lose the weight. In today's economy, that's over $700! She really did want the best for me and tried the only way she knew to motivate me to be skinny—her version of healthy. So back I went to a new kind of diet bars and diet drinks. I starved my way back down to 105 pounds.

I kept my weight between 105 and 120 pounds throughout high school. The actual number on the scale depended on how many diet pills I was taking and how obsessive I was about exercising. I actually made it all the way down to 95 pounds for two weeks by taking diet pills three times a day and not eating. Professionals never diagnosed me, but it's hard to argue that I didn't have an eating disorder. I just saw it as everyday life.

After high school, I maintained 120 pounds until I got married. I weighed in at 118 pounds on my wedding day. I was sure that weighing below my perfect weight was a good omen. While the number on the scale seemed to be a good weight for me, I wasn't healthy, nor was I eating in a healthful manner. However, "healthy" didn't exist in my world at that time—only "skinny."

After 24 years of marriage, five miscarriages, four babies, and a life of trying to pretend everything was good, I really did balloon. I didn't know it then, and it wasn't until years later that I would even admit to myself that my childhood had included sexual abuse and I had chosen a high-conflict, controlling marriage.

The weight gain was slow at first. I started by adding a few pounds, just six weeks after the wedding. I would go up a bit, then lose a few pounds through self-hatred and starvation. I continued to force my body into famine on a regular basis. Dieting never really worked well again. Every time I lost some weight, I would gain all of it back . . . plus a little more. In the 1980s, this concept of weight cycling, better known as "yo-yo" dieting[2], was not commonly understood. Today we know that someone who goes on a restrictive diet is more likely to gain weight than to lose any weight and keep it off.

As the weight gain and self-loathing increased, my cycle of self-abuse continued. I consistently went on some major diet, lost most of the weight, and would keep it off for at least six months, sometimes longer. No matter how old I was, if I lost the weight, my mom rewarded me with shopping. My mother was intent on having me be little. She saw me as more valuable—and happier—if I were skinny. Again, she wanted the best for me, but just didn't know how to provide what I really needed, which was self-acceptance and self-love. No one but I could provide that. "Healthy" had never been a part of my life, either mentally or physically, and I was certain that she was right. If I were skinny, then I could be happy and all of my other problems would just disappear.

I continued to hide the truth of the high conflict in my marriage and deny and repress the sexual abuse of my teen years. I hid the truth from myself and then eventually, as I recognized the truth of my troubled childhood, I tried to hide it from others. I was unable to keep the weight off. Every time I would manage to lose a few pounds, I would always put the weight back on plus a little more.

Eventually I gave up. I convinced myself that my obesity was a product of my genetics and, of course, I didn't have a chance against that. I told everyone I was fine with my size. I wore cute clothes, wore my makeup beautifully, and always had my hair done. But none of this masked the pain I felt inside; it was only an attempt to hide it to the outside world.

I finally quit checking the numbers the day I stepped on the scale and it said 255 pounds. I just couldn't accept 255 pounds on my five-foot-four-inch frame. So I quit weighing myself.

Five months later (and most likely at least ten pounds heavier) my marriage finally imploded, I filed for divorce, and within three months I weighed 180 pounds. In six months I was down to 160 pounds and a year later I was down to 155 pounds. I had lost about 100 pounds. I knew that in order to manage life on my own while raising four children, I would have to become very strong in body, mind, and soul.

It was a process that didn't happen in just six months. This was the culmination of all the diets I'd ever been on and all the failed diets I had been on, which was the exact same number.

I had dieted so many times that I had learned the most important lesson of dieting: diets don't work. So I decided to try something else that I had heard about. It was very radical and I had never actually met someone who had done it and succeeded, but it made more sense than anything I had ever tried. It was the idea that I should eat when I'm hungry and stop when I am full.

I didn't have to count calories and I didn't have to count points. I didn't have to eat only one meal a day, or eat seven meals a day, or exercise twice a day, only eat bananas and grapefruit, never eat bread, always eat protein, or make sure every meal was balanced with 40 percent carbs, 40 percent vegetables and 20 percent protein. Or maybe it was 20 percent carbs, 20 percent vegetables and 60 percent carbs . . . I could simply trust my body to know what to eat. This is what I chose to do.

But what to eat was my question. If there were no rules or points or calories or instructions, how would I know what to eat? I wasn't sure. I only knew was that I was going to eat whatever I wanted and whenever I wanted it. For the first few months, the only food group I wanted was chocolate. And the only food in that group that I wanted was M&M's. So I began to eat when I was hungry and stop when I was full. Every day I ate M&M's when I was hungry and stopped when I was full. Occasionally, I drank a glass of wine. And the weight came off.

After about three months, my body adjusted and began to crave protein, fruits, vegetables, and other food groups my body needed to have for nourishment. I still ate when I was hungry and stopped when I was full as I listened to my body's needs.

I felt good. I was dancing (my favorite form of exercise) and all was right with the world. I had achieved a version of skinniness and I knew that *must* mean I was happy.

A year later, I met the most amazing man and we fell in love. We got engaged and started to plan our wedding. Then one day I woke up and had gained ten pounds back, and then a few months later it was 20 pounds and then 30 pounds.

Two years after my initial weight loss and only four months into my engagement, even though I *knew* I would never gain back the weight, I was back up to 180 pounds and climbing.

I had fallen back into the place of not honoring what I wanted and needed. I had allowed someone else to fill the place of acceptance and love, rather than giving it to myself. I had to make some tough life decisions to head back to myself as I was created to be. I chose to tell this beautiful man that I could not marry him. We were both sad, but I knew I had made the right choice.

I looked at my world and made the decision to take back my life. So much of my life had slipped away from me, and I had allowed it to happen again. Although there were many layers to this discovery of understanding weight loss, I realized the key was falling in love with my own life. When I started on the weight loss journey that was what mattered—not M&M's and wine or the divorce. The key was simply to love myself.

I had spent most of my life trying to get others to love me. Through the years I had chosen to put everyone else's needs before my own. Instead of loving myself and approving of myself, I needed the approval and love of others to feel good. If I didn't have that love, then I turned to food. Of course, it wasn't until years later that I began to learn that the more I felt "less than" the more I ate to make myself feel better or at least "as good as."

After I regained the weight I realized it was essential that I begin to celebrate my own life if I was going to get the weight off again. I began to write down amazing things that happened in my world. Some of them were as simple as the fact that the kids got off to school with clean socks; others were more traditional: work success, birthdays, holidays, etc. I began to celebrate my world and my place in it as I fell back in love with myself. The more I celebrated in real wasy, the less I needed to fill that space of celebration.

A year later, I had lost the 40 pounds that I had regained and I made the decision to confront the personal demons that had driven me to fill up my emptiness with food. I faced the trauma, the challenges, the joy, and the grief that we call life.

We move with life; we don't just go through life. It is always a process for me, and it will be for you. Each day is still an adventure in finding my authentic soul and living in my authentic body.

As you begin to discover the adventure and joy of your authentic body, being to find ways to celebrate the small changes in your life. Celebrating creates the awareness that life has more joy than you may have realized. As the joy becomes part of your life you will begin to fall in love with your life and that is the beginning of the change of everything else.

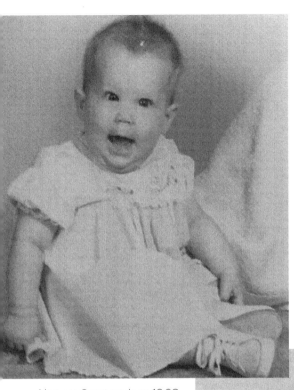

Above: September 1962. I was 9 months old and we had just moved into the house my father had built. He still lives in that house.

Right: December 1966. I am 4 years old. I only know this because I have no front teeth. The summer before I had fallen and all my front teeth were knocked out. I still remember the comfort of eating baby food bananas. This may have been the beginning of comforting myself with food.

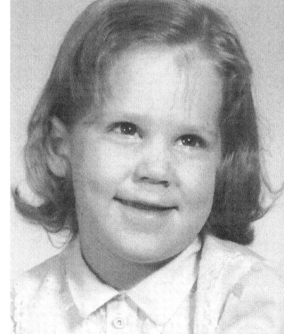

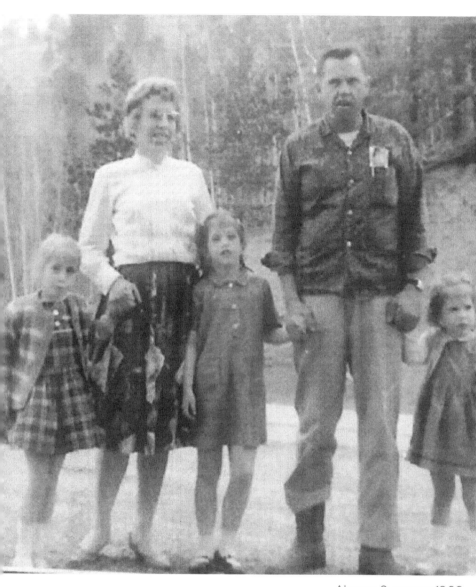

Above: Summer 1966.
With my Mom, Dad, and my
two older sisters in Palmer Lake,
Colorado. I am on the far right.
This picture—that I love—was my
mom's least favorite from that time
because she was at her heaviest
weight then. I always hoped I'd be
as beautiful as she was to me.

Below: Easter 1966.
This picture with my Mom and sisters is one of my favorites. I 'm just to the right of my mom. There are not many snap shots of our growing up years. In this picture each of us girls is posing exactly as we live life now. I'm just figuring out life and laughing along the way. This is the picture I used for years to remind myself of my authentic nature. Do you have one of yourself before the world told you who you should be?

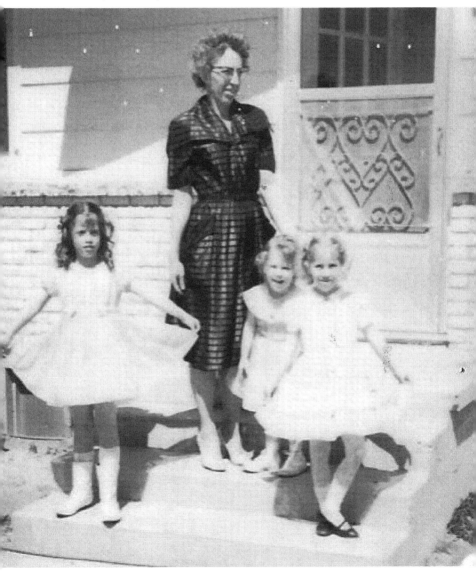

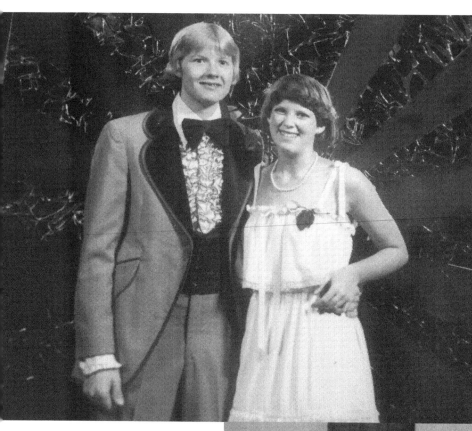

Above: Spring 1978. Prom with my first boyfriend. I had lost 25 pounds that spring and had done it mostly by starving myself. This sweet boy was so kind to me.

Right: Fall 1979 This was homecoming my senior year. My lifetime friends left to right Cathryn (Saunders) Karmondy, Valeria (Neale) Spencer, Jerri Craig, I'm in front. I maintained my weight that year through dieting, diet pills, and a fitness obsession.

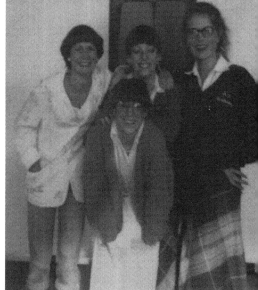

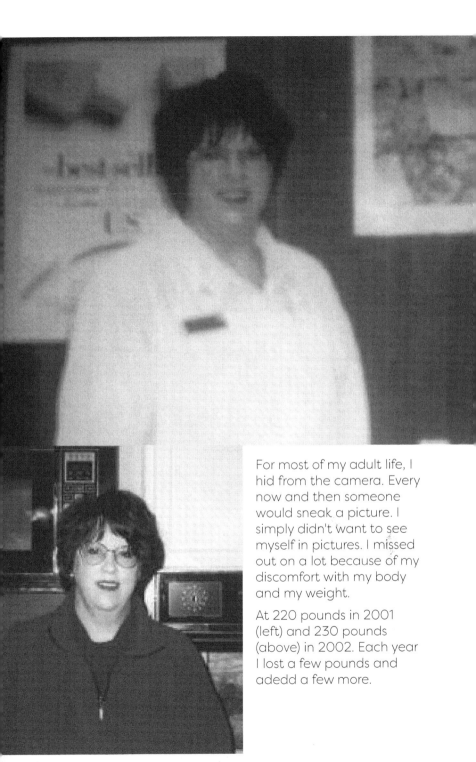

For most of my adult life, I hid from the camera. Every now and then someone would sneak a picture. I simply didn't want to see myself in pictures. I missed out on a lot because of my discomfort with my body and my weight.

At 220 pounds in 2001 (left) and 230 pounds (above) in 2002. Each year I lost a few pounds and adedd a few more.

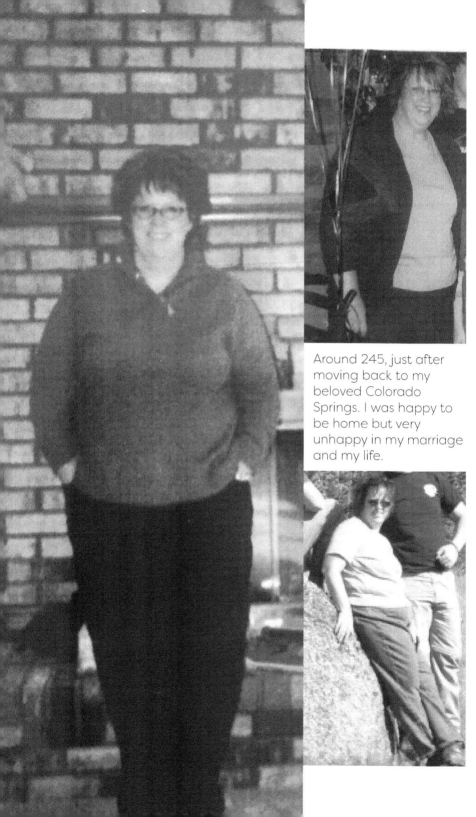

Around 245, just after moving back to my beloved Colorado Springs. I was happy to be home but very unhappy in my marriage and my life.

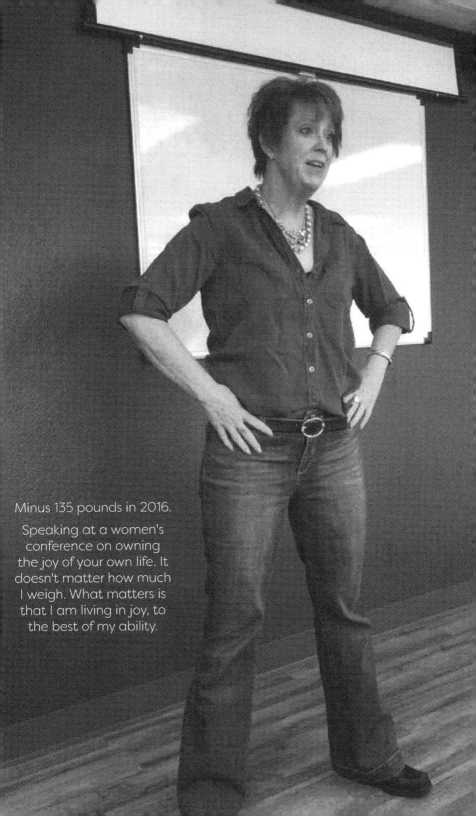

Minus 135 pounds in 2016.

Speaking at a women's conference on owning the joy of your own life. It doesn't matter how much I weigh. What matters is that I am living in joy, to the best of my ability.

Life with Soul Sisters is the only way to go.

Here's to Soul Sisters and the people we chose to do life with.

Top (from left to right): Anne Marlowe, Jessica Arent and me.

Bottom [from left to right] Cathryn (Saunders) Karmondy, Megan (Carroll) Miks, me, Valeria (Neale) Spencer. Forty plus years of friendship and we keep our stories to ourselves. These women have walked through life with me.

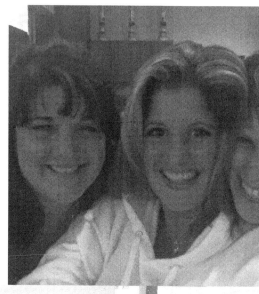

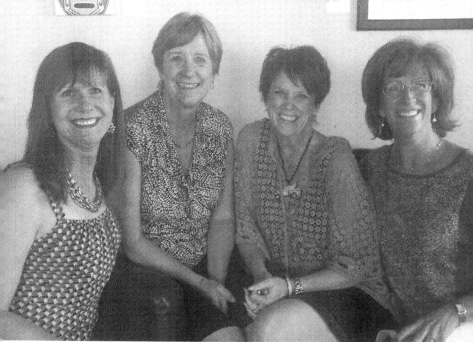

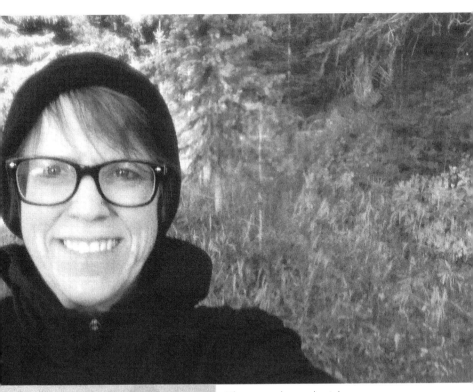

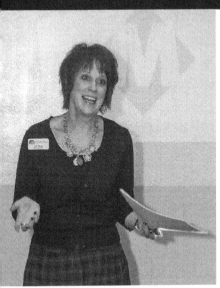

It's amazing what happens when you find joy.

Joy is simply about living in gratitude and embracing all the love around us.

Life is so much fun.

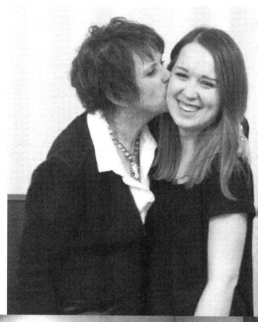

Top:
My daughter, my heart.
Gracie Packard and me.

Bottom:
My beautiful family.
My precious grand-
daughter Maggie
Valdez-Packard and her
beloved bear, Bo, in front.
Behind her is my second-
born son and her father
David Packard, me,
Gracie, Jacob Packard
(number three of the four)
and Mark Packard, my
oldest son. My father is in
the front.

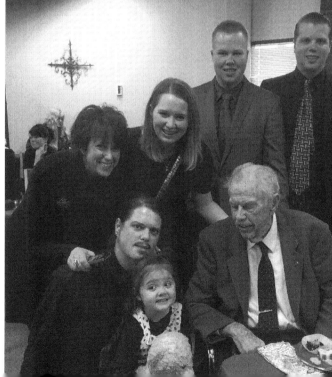

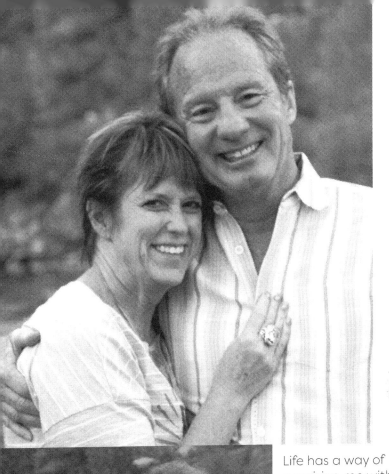

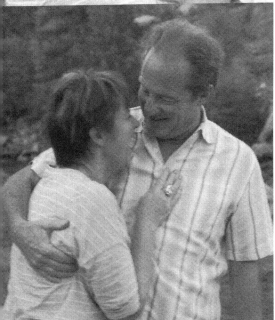

Life has a way of surprising me with joy as I keep moving forward with love. After years of being single, Jamie Fletcher showed up and made my life even richer. Learning to embrace all of life is a process, be gentle on yourself as you learn new skills to deal with life and love.

FINDING YOUR WAY
Fall In Love with Your Life (Example)

Use this journal as a way to start falling back in love with your life.

For the next week find three amazing things that happened each day or remember three amazing things about yourself. Write them down. Give yourself a party. Celebrate by doing something for yourself. It can be as simple as writing a great idea in the celebration section or as elaborate as taking yourself on vacation. It's your choice. Each day amazing things happen; when you recognize them you will begin to fall more deeply in love with yourself.

Three Amazing Things That Happened Today	Why It Was Amazing	How I Celebrated
I did the laundry and got it put away.	Everybody has been sick and I've been feeling behind.	Putting empty laundry baskets back in everyone's room.
Got a call from the editor of my book.	He sees good potential in it. He gave me a list of things I need to do next.	Called a good friend to tell her. Asked her to give a big "YES!" with me.
Everybody got their homework done before bed and without meltdowns.	We are finally moving into a routine after school started. The kids are starting to feel more comfortable with their course load. It gave me extra time to relax.	Chose to read an extra chapter of my book with the extra time I had available.

Download a printable worksheet at JillDavisCoaching.com/worksheets

FINDING YOUR WAY
Fall In Love with Your Life

Use this journal as a way to start falling back in love with your life.

For the next week find three amazing things that happened each day or remember three amazing things about yourself. Write them down. Give yourself a party. Celebrate by doing something for yourself. It can be as simple as writing a great idea in the celebration section or as elaborate as taking yourself on vacation. It's your choice. Each day amazing things happen; when you recognize them you will begin to fall more deeply in love with yourself.

Three Amazing Things That Happened Today	Why It Was Amazing	How I Celebrated

Download a printable worksheet at JillDavisCoaching.com/worksheets

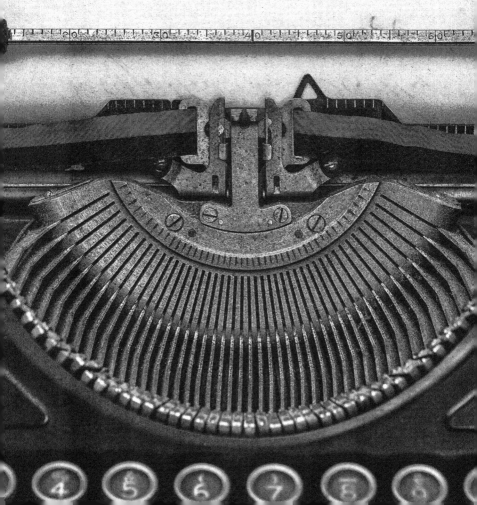

You must create a story of your life that is so compelling it propels you to your best life. Then no story of the past will be strong enough to stop you.

— Jill Davis

CHAPTER 2

*Who are we but the stories we tell
ourselves, about ourselves, and believe?*

— Scott Turow

OUR LIVES ARE THE stories we tell ourselves. The past is simply one of those stories, as is the future. We can actually change both of those stories. What we can't change are the facts. This is where we start to change our story.

We begin by recognizing the facts or data of our story and then deciding which story we want to write. The story we write eventually leads us to our ultimate result. If we want different results, then we must change the story.

Years ago, when I realized that the life I had been living was pretend and I didn't want to live it anymore, I began a deep study of trauma, cognitive therapy, and body work. I read as many self help books as I could get my hands on and I learned to listen to the Divine in a way I had never done before. I wanted to live authentically. I needed to become true to my life purpose. Through this process, I began to understand a very basic principle: I am the story that I write.

You are also the story that *you* write.

The best part of knowing and understanding that I am the story I choose to write is that I can always rewrite the story. The popular television show *Once Upon a Time* has an author who writes the stories of all the characters and he can change the plot, eliminate characters, and rewrite history as he chooses. Fortunately, we cannot do that to others' stories; but we can rewrite the story for ourselves.

When we rewrite the story, we can change the way we see the information and begin to change the outcome. It's how we see the situation, not what the facts of the situation are, which makes the difference in the end result. This also allows us to choose the outcome we want as we move forward in our lives and dreams. The story we tell can actually help us live in the body we were created to have.

Here is an example from my life:

Story 1:

I was born into a family of mental illness. I was the youngest child, but my mother lost a son to a stillbirth when I was two. She expressed the desire that if she could have chosen, she would have chosen the boy. My mother was not able to care for me in the way I needed. I was often forgotten and frequently neglected. My father struggled in the beginning of his career and finances were quite tight until my later years in high school. Oftentimes, there was not enough money for the lifestyle I needed to feel comfortable in my higher socioeconomic world of friends, so I constantly felt less than they.

Outcome of Story 1:

It creates a feeling of depression, victimhood, anger, blame, and disappointment, which results in inactivity and repeating the story for my children.

Story 2:

I was born into a family of mental illness. As the youngest child of several siblings, including multiple foster children, I was very fortunate to always have several playmates and friends at any time, day or night. I learned to be independent early on in life as my mother's mental illness did not allow her to provide some of the care I needed. Because I was often alone, I became a lifelong reader. Books became the friends I could always depend on. I learned to work hard and earn money early in life as I worked with my father while he was growing his business. Although many of my friends appeared to have more money and things than I did during childhood, I learned to value the worth of money and possessions and what it took to get them. This led to my strong work ethic and my desire to do the right thing with everything I have.

Outcome of Story 2:

I feel deep gratitude, joy, a sense of purpose, and the ability to embrace my life with a sense of belief.

Both stories start with the same fact: I was born into a family of mental illness. It's which story I tell after that statement that changes the outcome. When I choose to change the story, I can change the ultimate outcome of my life.

Now it's time for you to rewrite your story.

REWRITE YOUR STORY

I have combined several methods you can use to change your story from negative to positive. This will make it easier for you to rewrite your story.

Here is a simple formula that you can use to change the outcome of your story.

Start by documenting your Unhealthy Story:

1. Acknowledge the Data

Data is simply the facts of the situation. There are no descriptors, no judgments, and no preconceived expectations.

2. Story

This is where we start creating our story; the place where we begin to pass judgment on others and/or ourselves. Often this is where we create false assumptions, as well. This is our thought process and judgment about the kind of person who would allow or participate or create the information from the data. This is also where we can blame others for the situation and fall into victim mode. Recognizing our emotions here is essential to being able to rewrite the story we want.

3. Action

We take action based on the emotions and beliefs we have about the story.

4. Outcome

Our actions, which are based on our story and how we feel about our story, create our outcome.

Sometimes it may seem that the story, with its emotions, is the data, but always remember that data is just information.

Once we understand how the outcome is impacted by the story, it becomes time to change the story. One way to help change the story is by questioning it.

Ask yourself questions like:

- Is this true? Sometimes a story can be perceived as truth based on our assumptions of behavior. The only truth is the data and as such the data is valid or invalid.

- If it's not true, I need to document the truth. If it is true, do I want to change the outcome?

- Why would I choose to think these things about others or myself?

- How does it serve and support me to believe this story?

- Why do I want this story to be true? (Sometimes it's about feeling comfortable with and moving beyond our failures.)

It's also important to decide what our desired outcome is. Do we want the outcome we have obtained or do we want a different outcome? Once we know our desired outcome, we can work backward to change the story and then we reach our desired outcome.

Now reverse the steps to write your Healthy Story:

1. Desired Outcome

2. Action

3. Story

4. Data

In the following unhealthy and healthy example stories, you can see how the data does not change, but everything else changes based on the story we tell ourselves. Most importantly, the outcome changes as you change your feelings and actions.

Create a story of the future that is so compelling that no story of the past can stop you. Change your story, change your actions, and you will achieve your desired outcome.

FINDING YOUR WAY
Unhealthy Story (Example)

Data	*I am 50 pounds overweight.*
Story	*What kind of person would allow herself to become 50 pounds overweight? I am not a good person. I am stupid and lazy. I should have been more disciplined. I'll never feel good about myself.*
Actions	*I am stupid and lazy; therefore, there is no point in making an effort I'll never lose this weight, so I won't even bother to try. Where's the ice cream?*
Outcome	*Because I feel stupid and lazy, I choose to continue to eat past full and lot listen to my body. I am depressed and filled with self-loathing.*

Download a printable worksheet at JillDavisCoaching.com/worksheets

FINDING YOUR WAY
Healthy Story (Example)

Outcome (Desired)	*Feeling comfortable in my skin. Feeling energy to keep up with my life. Feeling strong and beautiful.*
Actions	*Brainstorm ideas to generate changes. Look at different ways to be aware of my hunger and fullness signals. Talk to people who are resources and can help me think differently. Start taking the steps to strengthen my body.*
Story	*I am a really smart person who is overweight. I want to get strong. I am determined and very disciplined. I will do what it takes to create the strong and healthy body I deserve. I will move toward the goals and desired outcome I want.*
Data	*I am 50 pounds overweight.*

Download a printable worksheet at JillDavisCoaching.com/worksheets

FINDING YOUR WAY
Unhealthy Story

Data	
Story	
Actions	
Outcome	

FINDING YOUR WAY
Healthy Story

Outcome (Desired)	
Actions	
Story	
Data	

It's amazing what happens when you learn you can eat anything at any time. You will stop wanting to eat everything all the time.

— Jill Davis

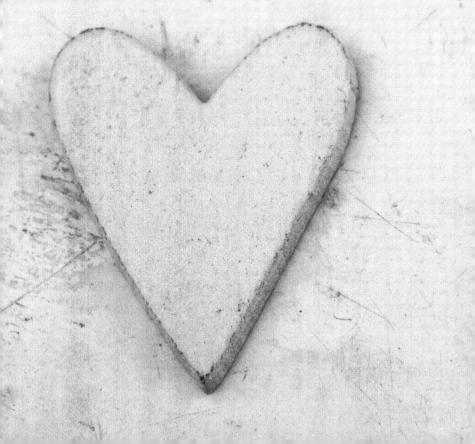

CHAPTER 3

Trust yourself.
You know more than you think you do.

— Dr. Benjamin Spock

OW MANY TIMES HAVE you gone to bed thinking, "How could I have had such a bad day?" How many times have you woken up thinking, "Today I am going to be *really* good?"

Most often when we think these thoughts, it's based on what we ate that day or what we plan to eat the next day. Somehow—through society, our own choices, our fears, or our thought processes—we have forgotten how to simply enjoy our foods and how to listen to our bodies.

When I had my first child, I was a very young mom and had no idea what to do with that surprising creation. There was no Internet, so no Pinterest, no "mommy at home" blogs, and no podcasts on raising children.

I only had my wonderful, old-timey, practical, Oklahoma-born pediatrician and my copy of the wonderful book by Dr. Benjamin Spock, *Baby and Child Care*. Although much of what they taught me back then would be considered out of date by our current standards, they both believed in child-directed parenting or at least for what was applicable at the time.

Dr. Spock was one of the first pediatricians to publicly state that children should be seen and not only heard. He also taught that children would not be spoiled if we held them when they cried. So simple today and so radical back then.

Both my pediatrician and Dr. Spock taught me that if I provided a variety of foods, my son would, over a period of time, choose the foods that he needed. I was grateful for this as I did not want to transfer my eating issues on to my children.

Our bodies crave nutrition, so they will crave the foods that we need. Our bodies know best, but with time and experience we learn how to override our natural instincts and end up making less-than-ideal nutrition decisions.

When I weighed 265 pounds, I was never hungry and never full. I needed nutrition, but I filled my body with food that did not contain the nutritional content I needed. My body could not understand what to do next. This is common for people who weigh more than their bodies are designed to weigh.

It may be that you haven't felt hungry in many years. Because we don't stop eating, we get frustrated with our overeating and decide we have bad moral character. We will continue to crave food until we meet our nutritional needs. Hunger and cravings are two different things.

Learning to eat simply to provide nourishment to our bodies is often referred to as intuitive eating. When children are provided a sampling of healthy foods they will intuitively know what to eat and how often. Children intuitively know what to eat and how often to eat.[3] In my opinion, as parents, we often teach them how not to eat intuitively by providing highly processed sugars too early and insisting on clean plates or a variety of foods.

In *The Common Sense Book of Baby and Child Care*, Dr. Spock wrote[4] that a parent "can trust an unspoiled child's appetite to choose a wholesome diet if she serves him a reasonable *variety and balance of those natural and unrefined foods which he himself enjoys eating at present* [emphasis added] even more importantly, it means that she doesn't have to worry when he develops a temporary dislike of a vegetable."

I believed Dr. Spock and I still do. You know yourself; you know what to eat and how much. Even though I started my weight-loss adventure with eating only M&M's, it wasn't long before my body began to crave more balanced meals. I could no longer live on nothing but chocolate and wine.

As you follow this process, you will learn what to eat and how much your body wants, and it won't be long before you don't have to be as aware. You will be able to eat anything you want, as long as you listen to your body.

Your Body has a Fuel Gauge

Learning to understand hunger signals is like learning to read the gas indicator on your car. It's easy, but you have to pay attention. A car will keep running until the last of the gas is gone. The car will sound the same until it stops running from lack of fuel. If you don't watch the gauge, there will be no other indicators that you need to refuel the car.

I learned about fuel gauges, and the importance of paying attention to them, early in my driving career. When I first started driving, I did not have a fancy car. I had a 1963 Rambler. I loved that car. It was from the days before seatbelts were mandatory and we could pack about ten high school students into it—more if there were some cozy couples! It took us on so many adventures and, as I recall, the speedometer went all the way to 120 mph.

The best part about the car was that it was a gift and my dad's company handled all the insurance, gas, and mechanical repairs. I had access to the company mechanic, whom I could call if I had problems with the car. He would get the car and fix whatever the problem was. This was a great benefit, but it didn't provide me with a working knowledge of how to keep a car running.

One day after school as I was looking for a place to get a snack, my car suddenly quit! I had no idea what to do so I called Joe, our mechanic. I was convinced my car was about ready to explode and I would die on the side of the road. (I was a bit of a melodramatic teenager.)

Joe came to rescue my car and brought the tow truck to take it across town to his shop. When he got in to start it, he burst out laughing. My car that was having "serious engine problems" was simply out of gas.

That's how we often are with our bodies; we ignore the fuel gauge for our body and then we mistake the feeling of hunger for a major physical emergency. We don't know what to do when our nutritional tank is empty.

Learn to Know Your Body Fuel Gauge

The first step is to recognize hunger, and then learn to eat when you are hungry and stop when you are full. It's very simple, but it's not easy. The beginning of identifying true hunger and fullness is becoming aware of what it feels like to be hungry.

1. Feeling Hunger

Remember a time you were really hungry, maybe after you had gone on a long hike or spent the afternoon swimming at the ocean. It is that feeling of real hunger and your body's need for nutrients. Find that time where it was not just a craving for sugar or carbs or emotional replacements, but a time when you were just really hungry and your body needed fuel. This is "running on empty" on your body's fuel gauge. It could also be called your body fuel gauge. When your fuel gauge feels empty, you are at a one on the body fuel gauge.

2. Feeling Full
Think about what it feels like to be really full. The feeling of full you have after Thanksgiving dinner or the 4th of July BBQ. This is the overflowing of your body's fuel tank. This feeling of not being able to take another bite is a ten on the body fuel gauge.

3. Be Mindful of Your Hunger
Start understanding your hunger feelings by being intentional before you eat anything and decide where you are on the hunger scale. Our bodies operate best when we don't get hungrier than a four and we don't eat till we are fuller than a six. Once you recognize the feeling of four on your personal body fuel gauge, it's time to eat.

4. Eat Only Until You are Full
Now begin with just a few bites. Take your time and find the place where your hunger is satisfied but you are not overly full and not beyond six on the body fuel gauge. As you learn to feel satisfied you will most likely begin to notice that the food stops being tasty at some point. This is a great indicator that you are getting to the place of fullness.

Typically the amount of food to start with is one quarter of your regular portion size. If you don't feel full after a quarter of your normal portion, then eat a little bit at a time until you feel satisfied. If you are not sure whether you are truly full, set aside the remaining food. Then when you feel hungry again, go through the same process.

While this may seem extreme, realize that most of us have forgotten what a "full portion" looks like and we no longer recognize the experience of satiety. We live in a food culture that wants more and believes that bigger is better (at least when it comes to portions). However, for our bodies, just enough really is perfect.

This process will help you retrain your body. Eventually you will remember what it feels like to go from hungry to full and begin to judge the amount of food you need to put on your plate to accurately fulfill your body's needs.

When you first start this practice, I recommend you begin by serving yourself your normal portion size on a plate. Then remove three fourths of the portion from the table or from view. This way you are able to focus on your hunger and fullness signals more consciously while not worrying about how to stop eating. The rest of the food is there for whenever you want it, and your body will tell you when and if you need it.

Use the body fuel scale at the end of this chapter as you learn to gauge your physical hunger. In time, you will instinctually remember what it feels like to be hungry and also what it feels like to have enough food.

It's Important to Trust Yourself Again

Learning to listen to both your hunger and fullness signals is a process in which you will learn to trust yourself again. As you have dieted, you have been told what, when, where, and how much to eat. You have been told—and have accepted—that you cannot trust your body to truly know what is best for you.

Learn to trust yourself. Trust will allow you to understand and love your body as you begin to release your no-longer-needed extra weight.

The relationship to your body is similar to a relationship between to intimate partners. When one or both partners have broken marriage vows through infidelity, it is very difficult to rebuild trust.

The only way that has been proven to build trust again is by really learning to listen to your partner as they talk about their feelings and emotions. This is true with your body as well. You have not been listening to what it is telling you.

In many ways you have been unfaithful to your beautiful body. You may have cheated on a diet, or had a cheat day from your diet. Either way, you have created a thought process that does not allow you to have full trust in your ability to know what and when to eat. The word cheat means to "act dishonestly or unfairly in order to gain an advantage". When we use the concept of cheating on ourselves we can interpret that to mean we are acting dishonestly with our bodies. It is a thought process that predisposes that we are not trusting ourselves.

To rebuild trust, you have to tune in to the truth your body is providing for you. Listen for your body's hunger and fullness signals and then honor them by only eating when you are hungry and choosing to stop eating when you are full.

Many years ago there was a trend amongst perpetual dieters. With each new diet they would lose some weight, then as soon as they stopped following "the plan," they would gain it back. This was when the concept of yo-yo dieting[5] was just beginning to be researched.

So a new "diet" concept became very popular. This new idea was to allow ourselves to eat only whenever we felt our stomachs growl. In some ways, it was a first step to a diet that allowed us to listen to our bodies' physical needs. But one of the problems with this specific concept is that a growling stomach is not typically an indicator of hunger.

According to the International Foundation for Functional Gastrointestinal Disorders, Inc., the growling sound in our stomachs is actually just air moving through our intestinal system.[6] It is often caused by over consumption of sugar, sucrose, fructose, or artificial sweeteners. The "growl" is not a good indicator of our hunger.

In the end, we learned another diet technique that wasn't effective. Sadly, this is a technique that many long-term dieters still adhere to. It's best to listen to our true hunger signals.

Why do we need to move beyond diets? Diets teach us to ignore our hunger and fullness signals. Diets tell you to eat at specific times even if you are not hungry and to eat the entire portion of a food, even if you are feeling full. These behaviors are deeply entrenched in our thought process and our body memory. It can take time to unlearn this behavior.

Food and Emotions

You will also have to differentiate between emotional hunger and physical hunger. Overeating is a form of self-medicating. We use food to deal with our emotions.

We come into the world with our body, mind, and soul connected. We know when we are hungry and we know when we are full. We eat because we need nutrition. However, it doesn't take long before we learn to equate food with love.

Our primary caretaker feeds us and we begin to associate food with getting our emotional needs met (or not met). Within a few years, we know if we are good we will get a cookie and if we are bad we will have to skip dessert.

That is one of the ways that food is used as a replacement for emotion. We take this conditioning of filling our emotional needs with food into our adult life. When we feel an emotion, we will often soothe the emotion with food consumption.

It may seem as if it should be simple to differentiate between emotional hunger and physical hunger, but it's not. When we lose the ability to recognize our physical hunger and fullness signals, we begin eating to satisfy emotional hunger; it becomes a habit. Now is the time to unlearn that habit, and the best way to do that is to start becoming aware of the symptoms of physical hunger and emotional hunger.

During my years of obesity, I knew I was an emotional eater but didn't know what to do about it. I had four children in 13 years. I was a homeschool mom. I was the spouse of a military commander. I volunteered for several organizations. I ran a successful direct-sales business with over 150 team members. I was a soccer, basketball, music, dance, and theatre mom. In many ways I was very successful and yet emotions continued to drive my overeating; so no matter how successful I was on the outside, I still felt like a failure on the inside.

I would get up in the morning and get breakfast for the kids, always something simple, but I wouldn't eat because I was going to be good that day. I had planned snacks throughout the day for the kids. These snacks were chosen specifically to provide good nutrition and happy tummies. I took care of their bodies and ignored mine. Dinner was either a freezer meal we had prepared earlier or fast food while we were running from one event to another.

We were a typical family, living in a small military town, trying to do the best we could. Watching my activity with my children and my family, you might wonder how I got so fat. However, I had a secret: I ate when no one was watching, and I ate a lot!

On the outside, everything looked perfect, but on the inside it was much less than perfect. I was in a lonely and difficult marriage and had not dealt with the trauma of growing up in a mentally ill family. Food was my one constant friend and companion and had been since I was a teenager.

Food helped to soothe the loneliness and gave me a private way to celebrate the good times. I ate when I was angry, when I was sad, when I was excited, when I was worried, when I wanted to celebrate, when I wanted to grieve, and just about any other time that I had an emotion. I worked hard to keep my emotions numbed and I used food to self-comfort.

I knew that I overate. I knew that I ate for emotional reasons and yet I had no idea how to stop. I had no idea that there was a way to learn to understand my emotions and move away from emotional eating. I was in such pain at the time. My main objective then was to stop the feelings. I had actually used food for so long, I didn't even realize I used it to stuff down my emotions until much later.

As I began my weight-loss journey, I simply wanted to get healthier and stronger. I didn't really care about why I was unhealthy. It wasn't until a few years later when I started to regain the weight and needed to take it off for good that I started looking at the "why" of my overeating.

When I lost the first 100 pounds, I did not take responsibility for my overeating and I blamed everyone else.

- If I had been nurtured and loved differently as a child, I wouldn't have gotten so fat.
- If I had been supported to choose college and a career, I wouldn't have gotten so fat.
- If I had just been given _____ (fill in the blank), I wouldn't have gotten so fat.

I believed all of that and much more, and eventually I started gaining the weight back. When I hit a 40-pound re-gain, I took a deep breath. I didn't want to be fat again, I didn't want to be in that painful place of beating myself up all the time, and most importantly I didn't want to lose the self-identity and self-worth I had worked so hard to recover. It was time to figure out why I ate the way I did.

I learned how to recognize the emotions that made me want to overeat before I actually overate. I learned to recognize and honor my feelings. I learned to feel my emotions, instead of eating them away.

It is actually very simple, but again, not easy, to learn how to recognize emotional eating. It takes time and awareness. Instead of continuing to diet, it's time to figure out what emotions are driving your eating.

Moving Beyond Emotional Eating

Until you take the time and learn to understand your emotions and why you overeat, you will continue to use food to soothe your emotions. I asked myself all the time when I was obese, "Why did you eat that?" I was finally in a place where I could understand which emotions created my overeating.

Now is your time to stop overeating for emotional reasons.

There are neurotransmitters released in our brains that create the feel-good emotions we all want and crave. It's why a one-year-old is unsure of eating a messy birthday cake, but after one taste, the same child realizes that sugar is amazing!

The desire for an artificial increase in these neurotransmitters is why we have a culture that tells us that if we are depressed, a serving (or two or three or more) of ice cream will make us feel better. When we eat carbohydrates, our brains release additional serotonin so we feel better.[7] This is how we learn to self-soothe with food.

We crave carbohydrates and other easily consumed foods to make our emotions either go away or to feel better. This is stuffing our bodies to avoid dealing with our emotions.

Overeating allows you to numb the emotions that you don't want to feel. According to researchers at the Institute of Neuroscience and Psychology at the University of Glasgow, there are four basic emotions. These emotions are mad, sad, glad, and afraid.

I learned that each of these emotions creates a specific type of eating. If you are not eating for physical hunger, you are eating for emotional hunger.

To learn to manage your emotions through behavior, you will want to start journaling them. I'm not suggesting you keep an intense, deep feelings journal, unless you want to. Just create a notebook or add a note on your phone documenting the times you eat and what it feels like.

The English language has so many words that describe the four basic emotions, so I created the feelings chart at the end of this chapter. It includes many descriptors for each emotion to help you better understand what you are feeling. As you begin to pay attention to each emotion you have when you eat, you will discover that you crave certain foods for certain emotions.

When we experience emotional hunger, we need to embrace the emotion and move through it. When we experience physical hunger, we need only to nourish our bodies.

Journaling your emotions and eating will help you to compare your emotional and physical hunger. Over time, you will begin to recognize these feelings without needing to be hyper vigilant. However, to start reclaiming your innate knowledge, you will need to be more aware of your emotions again.

The Truth About Good Food and Bad Food

Accepting that you can eat any food you want is a difficult concept for so many of us who have negative concepts of food. We are taught what to eat, when to eat, how to eat, and why not to eat. We are taught which foods are good and which foods are bad. Over time, we learn that we are good if we eat only certain foods that have been deemed "healthy" at that moment. Then we begin to believe that we are bad if we overindulge in certain foods that are considered to be bad for us.

If you don't quite understand this concept, I want you to think back to the last time you were at a party that had a buffet table with an assortment of foods: carrot sticks, roast beef, cheese trays, wings, chips, salsa, guacamole, salad, a variety of breads, butter, cookies, cheesecake, fruits, etc.

Did you look at that table and think, "I've been eating too much this week. I need to be really 'good' tonight"? Or perhaps you thought, "Oh well, I was really careful today in what I ate. I only ate a little salad and a diet shake—I deserve those cookies." Perhaps you thought, "Well, I have no willpower. I'm just going to give up and eat (meaning overeat) whatever I want. I can't help being bad."

In moments like those, you may believe that you are truly a good or bad person intrinsically, based on the foods you consume.

Food is not good or bad, and you are not good or bad based on what you eat. You are who you are and you have eaten a food because you ate it, simply that. You are of high value regardless of what food you eat to fuel your body.

As you move into honoring your body, begin to appreciate that you were created with taste buds. Food will become delicious, yummy, satisfying, nutritious, enjoyable, beautiful, and interesting instead of just being good.

You may not like every food, but there is no "bad" food or "good" food. Food has no morality. It simply is an object. While you are learning to trust your body, begin to enjoy your food again. Choose foods you love to eat, choose foods that bring you joy. In time, this is the only type of food you will eat. You will learn to trust yourself again and fall in love with food that beautifully nourishes you.

BODY FUEL GAUGE
Eat when you are hungry.
Stop when you are full.

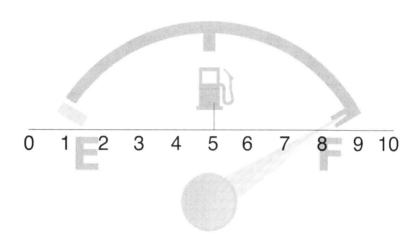

Optimal Range is Between 4 and 6

0 = Starving; feeling desparate; headache; very irritable

2 = Need to eat something; hunger pangs; somewhat irritable

4 = Somewhat hungry; stomach feels empty

5 = Neutral; neither hungry or full

6 = Satisfied; comfortable

8 = Uncomfortable; overfull; sluggish

10 = Stuffed; "Why did I eat so much?"

Download a printable worksheet at JillDavisCoaching.com/worksheets

Emotional	Physical
Emotional hunger comes on suddenly. There are no physical warning signs. There are just immediate feelings of hunger and cravings.	Physical hunger comes on slowly. You start feeling the effects of being hungry before you get to the place of needing to eat.
Cravings are specific. Nothing will stop the hunger except the particular food you crave.	Hunger is non-specific. You can look at a variety of choices and several options feel acceptable.
Emotional hunger is mind and mouth hunger. You will think about the food and decide how to get it. You may obsess on it till you obtain it.	Physical hunger is based in the body. It might be a stomach rumble, a feeling of emptiness, a slight headache, or even a feeling of being grumpy.
Emotional is demanding. It won't wait and wants immediate gratification.	Physical is patient. It knows that you have the reserves to move through hunger.
Emotional hunger is just that—emotional. It happens when you are mad, sad, afraid, or glad, and you use it to slow down or numb the emotion. Often you don't recognize it when you start and only become aware of it after you have overeaten.	Physical hunger comes from true physical need. Your body needs to be nourished and recognizes your need for nutrition. Typically happens after four or five hours since the last time you ate. Refer to the body fuel gauge to help you learn to feel physical hunger.
It often occurs as mindless eating. You don't notice until you realize you've eaten the whole bag of M&M's. This can also be social when we eat to connect with others.	It is conscious eating. You are aware of what you are putting into your body and why you are eating it. You choose how much or how little to eat and when you want to eat it.
Emotional eating goes past the feeling of full.	Physical eating stops when you are full without have to put a mental stop on eating.
Creates guilt. You beat yourself up and say all sorts of bullying words to yourself both during and after eating.	Knows that eating is part of life. You eat to live not live to eat.

Based on the cumulative teaching by Doreen Virtue, PhD on compulsive and binge eating. See reading list for further information.

FEELINGS CHARTS

Glad		
Alive	Great	On top of the world
Blissful	Gregarious	Over the moon
Content	Passionate	On cloud nine
Joyful	Compassion	Grinning from ear to ear
Joyous	Calm	Friendly
Delightful	Close	Marvelous
Delighted	Cherished	Warm
Contentment	Happy	Trusting
Excited	Wonderful	Happy camper
Excitement	Proud	Jumping for joy
Enamored	Loved	Lighthearted
Free	Confident	Tickled pink
Exhilarated	Hopeful	Pleased
Glowing	Kind	Radiant
Euphoric		Optimistic

Mad		
Annoyed	Defensive	Wounded
Bitter	Uptight	Up in arms
Indignant	Jealous	Sore-headed
Irate	Contemptuous	Black-mooded
Irritable	Grumpy	Fit to be tied
Offended	Hateful	Agitated
Exasperated	Critical	Perturbed
Resentful	Self-Loathing	Smoldering
Enraged	Mean	Worked up
Displeased	Hot-headed	Vengeful
Fuming	Seething	Ticked off
Infuriated	Spiteful	Disgusted
Frustrated	Violent	Unforgiving
Tense	Cross	Vindictive
	Cruel	

FEELINGS CHARTS

Sad		
Abandoned	Tearful	Forsaken
Abused	Unimportant	Pessimistic
Alone	Worthless	Sorrowful
Lonely	Unloved	Slighted
Blue	Vulnerable	Crushed
Gloomy	Withdrawn	Injured
Glum	Awful	Heartbroken
Helpless	Bleak	Offended
Downcast	Insignificant	Fragile
Empty	Used	Grieving
Inferior	Unfit	Sorrowful
Insecure	Unacceptable	Moody
Isolated	Lost	Despondent
Upset	Like a failure	Moros
Useless	Immobilized	Mourning
Weepy	Rejected	Melancholy
Suffering		Heavy-hearted

Afraid		
Threatened	Timid	Wary
Scared	Intimidated	Nervous
Fearful	Shocked	Intolerant
Apprehensive	Frightened	Self-hatred
Panicky	Alarmed	Combative
Startled	Shaky	Timorous
Terror-stricken	Edgy	Petrified
Horrified	Defensive	Trapped
Aghast	Bewildered	Helpless
Disturbed	Guarded	Confounded
Dismayed	Suspicious	Desperate
Daunted	Paranoid	Distrustful
Stunned	Aggressive	Bundle of nerves
	Attacking	

FINDING YOUR WAY
Food Journal (Example)

You can eat anything you want when you listen to your body.

Date					
Time	8:45 am	12:20 pm	3:00 pm	5:45 pm	8:00 pm
Hunger Scale Before	4	3	6	4	5
Hunger Scale After	5	5	8	6	7
Emotion	Busy, Centered	Life is good	Bored	Content	Happy
Food	Coffee, half & half, egg, tortilla, ground turkey, pepper jack	Egg, fajita tortilla, soy chorizo	Chocolate bar, bannan, and some grapes	Chicken brest grilled, black beans, cheddar cheese	Red wine, popcorn
Other					Movie with sweet-heart, having fun!

Download a printable worksheet at JillDavisCoaching.com/worksheets

FINDING YOUR WAY
Food Journal

You can eat anything you want when you listen to your body.

Date					
Time					
Hunger Scale Before					
Hunger Scale After					
Emotion					
Food					
Other					

Download a printable worksheet at JillDavisCoaching.com/worksheets

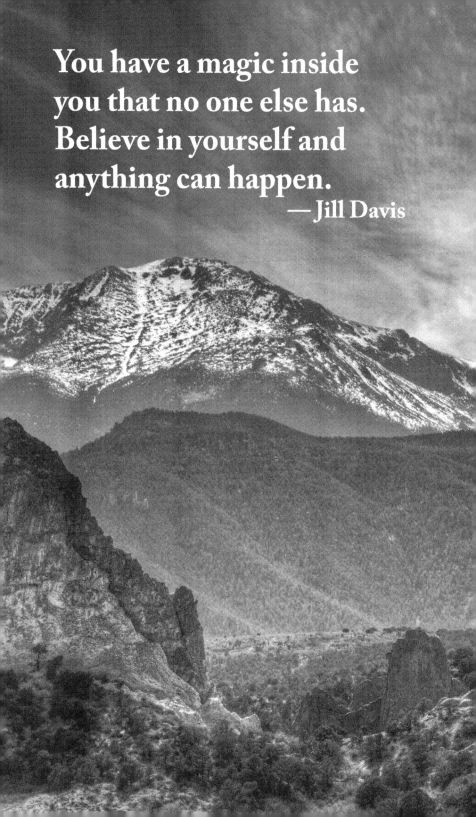

You have a magic inside
you that no one else has.
Believe in yourself and
anything can happen.
— Jill Davis

CHAPTER 4

Can you remember who you were, before the world told you what you should be?

— Danielle LaPorte

EVERAL YEARS AGO, **I** sat at the side of a water fountain and watched my beautiful six-year-old daughter dance, twirl, and spin through the water. She was fully conscious of her body and what it would do for her, but fully unconscious of what others thought of her. She wasn't thinking about how her belly showed, or whether her thighs were too heavy, of whether her swimsuit looked good on her. She simply loved the feeling of twirling, spinning, and dancing. I remember thinking if only all women could love their bodies the way we did when we were six.

I remember distinctly the first time I questioned whether my body was beautiful. It was the summer when I was ten. I grew up swimming, first at a little local park and then at the local country club. I started swimming for the swim team when I was six. I *loved* to swim. I *lived* to swim. It was my passion and my joy.

That summer, I started to go through an early puberty: growth spurt, hormonal changes and all. I wasn't quite aware that my body was going through a drastic change. In 1972, when I was ten years old, we didn't talk about those things much. But I knew I felt different and my body didn't feel quite like my own. I felt as if I was all elbows and knees. I was always running into something, bumping my toes and nose, and generally not feeling very comfortable in my own skin.

One day, after swim practice, I was running back to my mom. She smiled at me and told me how beautiful I was, then she said, "You will be a beautiful young lady, if you can keep from getting fat like your aunt."

These words brought awareness to me that I had never had before. I had never even thought about being fat or skinny—I just was a kid with a body.

Until that moment, my mind, body, and soul had been integrated. My aunt was well loved but also a constant source of conversation because of her obesity. Now I was afraid I would take on that role. It became important to me to have full mastery over the size of my body.

My mom wasn't trying to hurt me or create any problems. It just happened to be the perfect storm: my awareness of my body changing and my mom telling me I would be beautiful as long as I didn't get fat. In my ten-year-old head I knew that beautiful must mean *not fat* and I stepped out of loving my body and into abusing my body.

When did you first realize you didn't love your body? Perhaps it was a simple statement like the one my mom made. It might have been a bully on the playground who didn't fully realize the power of words. Maybe a picture of a beautiful model who looked so different than you did that you knew you must be flawed.

Whatever the reason was, now is the time to move back into loving your body.

Positive Body Image

Over the last few years, social media has been moving into the concept of body acceptance and positive body image. According to the National Eating Disorders Association[8]:

"Body image is how you see yourself when you look in the mirror or when you picture yourself in your mind. It encompasses: What you believe about your own appearance (including your memories, assumptions, and generalizations). How you feel about your body, including your height, shape, and weight. How you sense and control your body as you move. How you feel in your body, not just about your body."

A negative body image happens when we don't appreciate our body. A positive body image includes recognizing, respecting and, yes, even loving your body. There are days where you may feel awkward or uncomfortable in your skin. On those days it's even more important to show love to your body. You can reduce those negative thoughts and feelings as you create positive and accepting feelings about your body.

The majority of women in the United States expresses at least some negative body image. Some studies show that 91% of women either hate their bodies or are very dissatisfied with them. Forty percent of ten-year-old girls are either on a diet or thinking of going on a diet. This used to be more of a women's issue, but more and more men are feeling the same, and now statistically 60% of men are unhappy with their bodies.

I remember so clearly, so many times, looking in the mirror and saying, "I hate my body." I didn't even allow my children to say they hated someone and yet I spent many hours talking to myself about how much I hated my body, hated my fat, hated the way I looked. Changing your body image is not something that happens overnight. Just like changing our relationship with food, it takes time and focus to change the relationship we have with our body.

A Journaling Exercise

Look in the mirror and think of all the adjectives you can use to describe your body and who you are. Every day, think of more words and add them to your vocabulary. Each day spend time with these words. There will come a day that one or more of them will become the theme of your life and your body.

Getting ready in the morning can be one of the most difficult times of our day. We get into the shower and out of the shower, spend time putting on lotion, and often spend that time hating our body. Instead, create ideas and thoughts that express your love for your body.

Look at your body and remember all the good things it has done for you. Begin to contemplate all the good your body has done for you and all the pleasure you have received from your body.

Each day brings an opportunity to love and honor your body.

FINDING YOUR WAY
A Love Letter (Example)

Dear Brave, Beautiful Body,

Thank you. I am so grateful for all that you have done for me over the years. From being strong enough that I could dance as a little girl to the endurance you now have for a full night out dancing with friends. I love the shape of your hips that could only have come from carrying four incredible children all the way to their delivery. And yes, I love every one of the scars on your body. They remind me of the day each of those children came into the world through a C-section. How brave you were to allow that and to heal from it!

Your eyes and nose are beautiful. Remember the boy who first sang "Brown-Eyed Girl" to you? Remember how special you felt because he found a song about brown eyes when everyone you admired had blue eyes? Today I see not only the brown of your childhood, but the golden flecks that came with the wisdom of time. Your little nose is a button nose and is beautiful.

Strong feet, I love you!!! Thank you for taking me on so many adventures, for allowing me to go barefoot so that I can feel the sand of the beach, the water of the Colorado mountains, and the warmth of the ground in the summer garden.

You, dear body, have given me so much joy and pleasure. I give you hugs, love, and joy. I am grateful for you and your beauty that includes scars and delight, hope and future. Thank you for all that you have done for me for so many years.

With much love,
Jill

Download a printable worksheet at JillDavisCoaching.com/worksheets

FINDING YOUR WAY
A Love Letter

Dear Brave, Beautiful Body,

With much love,

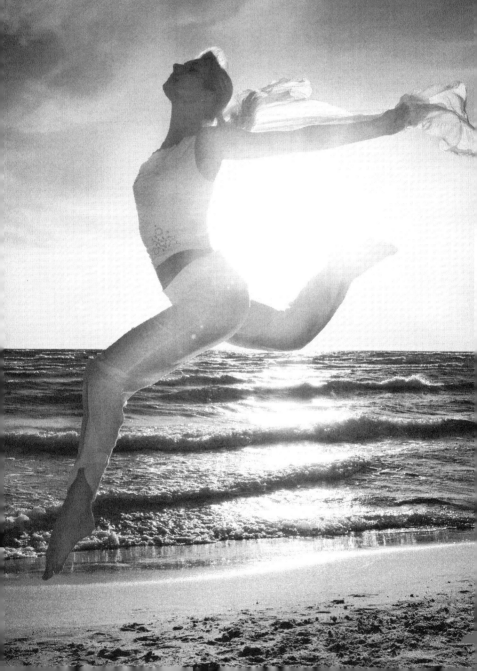

Sometimes you just gotta dance!
Dance into JOY! Move with JOY!
— Jill Davis

CHAPTER 5

We can never make peace with the outer world, until we find peace with ourselves.

— Dalai Lama

I AM AN OBSERVER OF people. I learned much about how to relate to others and how to get along with people from watching my siblings and my parents as I hid under the dining room table. I spent much of my childhood and adolescence fascinated about why people do what they do. I was delighted when I learned that philosophers and psychologists had wrestled with that very topic for thousands of years.

When I became a beauty consultant with Mary Kay Cosmetics, I learned about DISC behavioral theory. This was a theory from early in the 20th century that helped me to understand why others did what they did and more importantly, why I behaved the way I did.

It made such a difference for me in the way I saw myself and those around me that I wanted to learn more. Over the years, I read many different books on personality styles and became certified in different methods of understanding how people operate in life.

I began to teach the principles to my Mary Kay unit and I saw the impact it had on them as they learned to meet the emotional needs of their customers and team members. Both team production and profits increased dramatically. Unit members also improved communication and connection in their personal relationships.

Over time, I learned that everything we do is impacted by our personality styles. From intimate partner relationships to how we raise our children, to how we react when we encounter road rage and how we interact in our work place. It also impacts how we eat and exercise.

Lyndon Johnson said, "If we are to live together in peace, we must come to know each other." Understanding behavioral and personality styles is one of the ways we can come to know each other. When we understand what motivates others and ourselves, it creates a language and conversation that can reduce conflict and confrontation and improve connection and communication.

Have you ever opened a magazine and seen a quiz about any type of emotional behavior or taken a quiz that your friend posted on Facebook about what kind of friend you are? This is an example of behavior-based performance. All of these behavior-based models have been created because we want to know why we do things the way we do and, more importantly, why others behave like they do.

The hope is that we will learn more about others and ourselves so that we can live in our strengths, reduce our weaknesses, and create better relationships in both our personal and professional lives. Life is about relationships. Better communication creates better relationships.

Understanding DISC allows us to increase our communication skills, which allows us to improve all of our relationships. This includes our relationship with our bodies and ourselves.

Maybe you've heard of this concept, or you've played with the fun Facebook tests. Perhaps you have even have taken a behavioral profile. But did you ever wonder where it came from?

Over four thousand years ago, Hippocrates knew that people behaved in certain ways and that there were personality traits common to different groups. He believed that the fluids, or humors, in our bodies are what determined our behaviors. These four humors were yellow bile, black bile, blood, and phlegm and they were associated with the personality types known as Choleric, Melancholic, Sanguine, and Phlegmatic.

These terms are still used by some in the personality styles field and were made popular by Florence Littauer in her book *Personality Plus* and followed by her daughter, Marita Littauer's, book *Wired that Way*.

Throughout history, others have tried to explain and understand how people are wired. Empedocles introduced the concept of the elements of Earth, Air, Fire, Water, and the mixture of Love and Strife to explain personalities.

There are many different types of personality profiles including DISC, Myers-Briggs, The Enneagram, Color Theory, The Big Five, The Keirsey Theory, and more. There are also many pop-culture quizzes based in these and other theories. Some of these theories help us understand our behaviors; others help us understand our motivation. Both kinds are important.

William Marston, who was a contemporary of Carl Jung, wrote a book called *The Emotions of Normal People* in 1928. Although his book is very theoretical, it was the basis for the current behavioral style profile known as DISC.

Marston outlined the four themes of personalities. His concept was that people could be grouped into four basic personality styles based on actions and behaviors. He labeled them dominance, inducement, submission, and compliance.

Marston's theory was that people would behave in a manner consistent with their environment, demands, and expectations. He taught that a person's behavior would vary from situation to situation based on their core behavioral style.

Although there are many different profiles and assessments, DISC is one of the easier ones to understand and to quickly implement to improve your interpersonal and business communication skills.

Because it is four basic styles, it's easy to recognize your style and others' styles, and can bring instantaneous results for your life and business. Although we each have primary and secondary styles, we are each a unique blend of all four styles. There are as many blends of personalities as there are blends of colors in the rainbow.

DISC and other behavioral style instruments are not only a way to understand your personality, your strengths, and your weaknesses, but they also create a vocabulary that you can use to express ideas with those around you. It is not a label or an excuse for behavior. It is one way, of many, to help you grow and become more of who you were created to be. It is your gift.

Remember that DISC is not about labeling yourself or others. It is simply a way of creating vocabulary to improve communication and to understand ourselves better so that we can understand others better:

DISC QUICK RECOGNITION

DIRECTIVE Large Body Language Finishes Sentences Style: Power Suit Needs to be in Leadership Needs Support for Goals Accomplishments are #1	**INFLUENCING** Open Body Language Lots of Stories Style: Dress to Impress Needs Recognition Needs Support for Ideas Activities/Fun are #1
CONSCIENTIOUS Closed Body Language Cautious When Speaking Style: Classic/Matched Clothes Needs Facts Needs Support for Thoughts Organization/Education is #1	**STEADY** Relaxed Body Language Observes Before Speaking Style: Relaxed Needs Relationship Needs Support for Feelings Relationships are #1

TASK FOCUSED (left side) — **PEOPLE FOCUSED** (right side)

SLOWER PACED

The #1 Way to Recognize a Personality Style Without a Profile

Ask the Question: *"Will you please tell me about yourself?"*

DIRECTIVE:
Will talk about accomplishments, awards, and activities.

INFLUENCING:
Will tell you lots of stories and back stories.

STEADY:
Will talk about relasionships—kids, family, pets, friends.

CONSCIENTIOUS:
Will ask "What or why do you want to know?"

D Style = Directive
Ds have the gift of direction

★ **D** styles know where they are going; they see the big picture and are anxious to take the action needed to get there. They use direct and large body language and fist-pounding to make their point. They have a quick processing style and are fast decision makers. They tend to be self-confident and assertive. They are trustworthy and competitive, and they excel in emergencies.

★ They are fast-paced and action-focused. Projects energize them.

★ Based on research by PeopleKeys™, they make up 3% of the population.

★ A **D**'s greatest fear: being taken advantage of.

★ You might be a **D** if anyone ever told you, "Don't be so bossy," or "Slow down; I can't keep up with you."

★ If you are a **D**, the best tip for you: When answering voicemail or email, be sure to listen to the end of the message or read to the end of the email. With your fast action-taking skills, you may skip over some important information.

★ When communicating with a **D**, be sure to be aware of their time. Be sure to show up on time and end a meeting at the time promised. It's important to let the **D** do much of the talking. He or she will ask you what they want to know.

★ If you are a **D**, when communicating to others, do your best to slow down, really listen, and be sure to say please and thank you.

I Style = Influence
Is have the gift of entertainment

★ I styles bring excitement and entertainment to life. They use expressive body language and tend to be very "touchy/feely." They are storytellers and are energetic and approachable. They are curious, imaginative, and enthusiastic.

★ Is are energized by being around people and are relationship-oriented. They are fast-paced and people-focused.

★ According to PeopleKeys™, Is make up 11% of the population.

★ An I's greatest fear: loss of social recognition.

★ You might be an I if anyone ever told you, "Shhhh, don't talk so much," or "You are such a social butterfly."

★ Best tip for an I style: If you are in a group and someone interrupts your story, don't bring it back up unless asked. The others really don't want to hear it right now. You'll have lots of other opportunities to share your stories.

★ When communicating with an I, be sure to plan lots of time to listen. They want to tell stories and be heard. You will also want to keep the topics light and fun, if possible.

★ If you are an I, when communicating to others, listen for understanding, not just how to respond. Slow down and work to stay focused on the immediate conversation without planning what to say next, and remember not to interrupt.

S Style = Steady or Stable
Ss have the gift of comfort

★ The **S** style personality's calm demeanor brings comfort and peace to most situations. They are steady and balanced with relaxed or "laid-back" body language. They tend to communicate in a soft voice. The more comfortable an **S** style person is, the quieter their voice can become. They are extremely consistent and want to create harmony for others.

★ They are energized by peace and calm and are relationship-oriented. They are slower-paced and people-focused.

★ According to PeopleKeys™, **S**s make up 69% of the population.

★ An **S**'s greatest fear: Conflict or Confrontation.

★ You might be an **S** if anyone ever told you, "Don't be so lazy," or "You're not living up to your potential."

★ Best tip for an **S** style: Conflict and change do not always disrupt peace. It can be a great way to improve relationships.

★ When communicating with an **S**, be sure to keep a steady pace to your conversation and lower your voice to match their level. They typically prefer conversations about people rather than activities. Be prepared to do much of the talking when you are with an **S** and don't ask too many questions or an **S** may feel overwhelmed.

★ If you are an **S**, when communicating to others, be sure to speak loud enough to be heard. Be willing to step into a conversation before the end of it. What you say has value and others will want to hear you.

C Style = Conscientious
Cs have the gift of order

★ The **C** style personality's ability to see details allows them to bring order from chaos. They are focused and aware with closed body language and few hand gestures. They are good listeners and loyal friends. They are focused on looking for details and tend to share their ideas only when they feel they can contribute value. **C**s like to complete one project fully before moving to the next.

★ They are slower-paced and action-focused. **C** styles are energized by solitude.

★ According to PeopleKeys™, **C**s comprise 17% of the population.

★ A **C**'s greatest fear: Being wrong or making a mistake.

★ You might be a **C** if anyone ever told you "Don't be so controlling," or "Don't sweat the small stuff."

★ Best tip for a **C** style: Perfection is difficult to obtain. Allow yourself grace when you make a mistake. It's okay to be wrong, and in most cases, very few people will notice it.

★ When communicating with a **C**, be sure to use details and facts to support your discussion. If you are unsure of an answer, offer to find the answer and get back to them rather than give a "best guess" answer. Be sure not to ask too many personal questions as they operate on a "need to know" basis. Do not tell long stories.

★ If you are a **C**, when communicating to others, listen to their stories, pay attention to their emotions, and focus on accepting people right where they are.

Personality Styles and Exercise

For years, as an extremely overweight woman, I was told go to the gym, work out, and lift weights. My favorites were, "It's simple math, Jill. If you just burn more calories than you consume, you'll lose weight," and "When you feel like eating, go work out." If I liked to work out and sweat, I would not have weighed 265 pounds.

The truth is that I still don't like to work out. To me, when I hear the words "work out," I envision some guy at a bodybuilding gym who is super buff and works out two hours a day, keeps track of all his workouts and everything he eats. Blech! To me that type of work sounds awful. But I know now it's because I am an **I**-wired behavioral style. My personality style needs to have fun and to hang out with other people. A dance class or Zumba is the perfect form of exercise for me.

If you have spent years thinking "I *hate* to exercise" or if you use exercise to work off stress, you have experienced the impact your personality style has on your physical activity. Once you know your style, review the following exercise tips to find the best activities for your personality:

D Style Exercise Tips:

- **D**s use exercise to reduce stress. For a **D**, competition is one of the most important parts of life and of body movement. Whether you are competing with yourself or in individualized competitive sports like racquetball, handball, or tennis, you will be happiest if you can find a way to win.

- **D**s tend to be in leadership and are very busy. This busyness can keep you from finding movement that you love. If you want to stay busy and productive and this desire is keeping you from moving your body, consider listening to audiobooks while you work out, or scheduling your social commitments around being outside and walking.

- **D**s tend to be adventuresome, so also look for activities like rock climbing, sailing, sky diving, or deep-sea diving. These will fuel your desire for an adrenaline rush while allowing you to move your body.

- A **D**-wired personality is very action-focused. Don't overdo it when you first start.

- Track your workout schedule so you are competing with yourself and can get quick wins. Make sure your goals are activity-related and not results-based. **D**s can get frustrated and move on if they don't get quick results.

I Style Exercise Tips:

- **I**s prefer movement that includes socializing. Participating in intramural sports with your friends is a great way to create body movement and enjoy socializing.

- **I**s tend to love dance as a body movement. Most gyms now offer multiple classes such as Zumba, Barre, hip-hop, and even pole dancing. These are also fun for the **I** style as they can go dancing out with friends and enjoy even more body-movement benefits.

- **I**s like social activities and team sports.

- **I**s do best when they have a buddy to keep them accountable. So even if the treadmill sounds boring, it can become a lot of fun if you use the time to chat with a friend. Finding friends to work out with will change the "work" out to a fun play time with friends.

- Be sure to establish rewards as you complete your goals. **I**s do best when they have fun rewards for what may seem like boring goals.

S Style Exercise Tips:

- **S** styles prefer to work out with just a couple of friends and tend to avoid big groups.

- A great way for an **S** style to move their body but still be more on their own are classes like Pilates, spinning, and kickboxing. In these classes, there is not a lot of interaction with others, unless you desire it.

- **S** styles also do well with water sports such as swimming, rowing, and kayaking.

- The **S** style can really benefit from the use of a personal coach, as it involves a one-on-one, long-term, trusting relationship. The **S** style thrives on such relationship.

- **S** styles are typically caregivers. It may help to keep you moving if you remind yourself that if you are not healthy, you will not be able to care for others as well as you would like.

- As an **S**, you will want to find environments that make you feel comfortable and are welcoming to you.

- When you decide to set your goal, allow yourself to reach it in small steps. You really can eat an elephant one bite at a time.

- Begin with a simple routine and then expand it to help you achieve long-term goals.

- **S** styles have a strong need to stay in their comfort zone. Take just one step out of your comfort zone, then one more. Before you know it, you will have learned to love moving your body.

C Style Exercise Tips:

- **C**s like independent activities that take skill and precision.

- **C** styles like to keep track of details. Smartphone apps like My Fitness Pal will be of great help to you.

- **C** styles prefer skilled activities, such as golf, biking, or running. Set goals based on increasing your skill set and you will be able to stay focused.

- Focus on a future goal such as improving your handicap, running a marathon, or taking a long bike ride. Then design a specific tracking system to get you to that goal.

- You might want to create a spreadsheet or a checklist to keep track of the steps.

- **C** styles will sometimes not get started because they can't to do it right and there is a learning curve. Don't procrastinate for perfection.

Yoga for Every Style

Yoga is one activity that helps every body, and every style, learn to love to move.

- **D** styles love that they are in charge of their own workout.

- **I** styles love the group class.

- **S** styles love the relaxation at the end.

- **C** styles love the structure and the goal of getting it right.

And finally, if all else fails, just put your favorite music on loudly and dance!

What's Your Style? Take the DISC Assessment

Now that you know more about the four personality styles, do you have any clues about your own style? Take the Mini DISC profile at the back of the book to gain a basic understanding of your personality style (or use it to quiz your family and friends!).

If you'd like to get an in depth personalized report and learn even more about your style, visit JillDavisCoaching.com/store to purchase a DISC assessment.

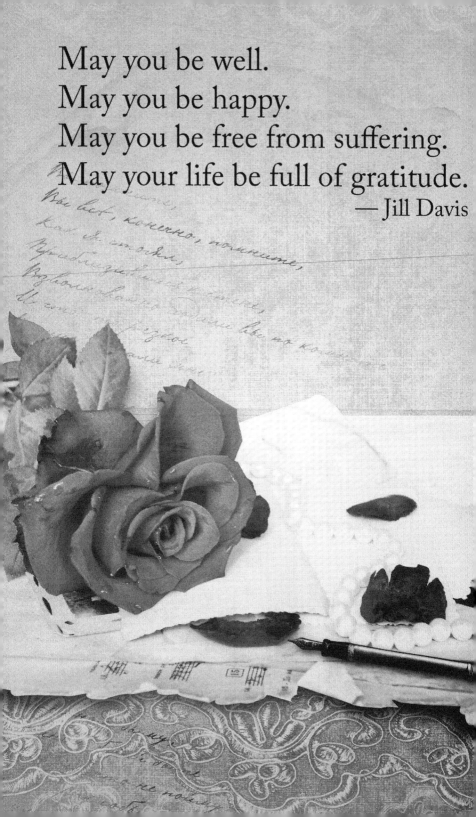

May you be well.
May you be happy.
May you be free from suffering.
May your life be full of gratitude.

— Jill Davis

CHAPTER 6

If the only prayer you ever say
in your entire life is "Thank you,"
it will be enough.

— Meister Eckhart

SHOWING GRATITUDE HAS BEEN a spiritual practice through the ages. All of the great masters have taught us to be grateful.

Plato said, "A grateful mind is a great mind which eventually attracts to itself great things."

Paul, the Apostle, said, "Give thanks in all things."

The Buddha said, "Let us rise up and be thankful, for if we didn't learn a lot today, at least we learned a little, and if we didn't learn a little, at least we didn't get sick, and if we got sick, at least we didn't die; so let us be thankful."

More recently, Sara Ban Breathnach teaches daily gratitude in her book *Simple Abundance*. Published in 1995, it is considered by many to be the beginning of the current gratitude trend.

On Instagram there is a "365 days of gratitude" section, where you can post a daily picture and a personal statement of gratitude.

Corrie Ten Boom, a survivor of the Nazi concentration camps, talked about being grateful for the fleas during her imprisonment, as they kept the camp guards away.

We know that being grateful changes our thought process as well as rewires our neural pathways. We can create new neural pathways—that lead us to compassion, gratitude, and joy instead of anxiety, fear, and anger.[9] UNC Berkley has done extensive research on how gratitude impacts our brains and our success for the better.

Years ago, my mother used to wake me up singing, "Count your many blessings, name them one by one." That was the beginning of my personal gratitude practice. I didn't actually think much about gratitude—it was just a part of my life.

Gratitude for a Change

Several years ago, I came to a place in my life where I knew I had to make significant changes. I had already changed my life radically by getting divorced and losing 130 pounds and yet there were still changes needing to be made. Although I had started the changes with much excitement, over a period of time I had become angry and bitter and blamed others for the fact that I had struggles. I could feel myself slipping into a place that I had never been before, a place where happiness and joy were elusive.

I didn't want to change, for I had become comfortable with my life, even in all its chaos. Yet I knew my soul would die if I stayed in that place. I was beginning to stuff my emotions again as I returned to overeating. I did not love my body, and was living in stress. Life was feeling out of balance and familiar all at the same time. It wasn't long, however, before the need for change overtook the want for the familiar. It has been said by many people in different ways that there comes a time when the pain of staying the same becomes greater than the pain of change. Then and only then will we choose the pain of change, which also is the joy of change. My pain pushed me into changing my life into a place of more joy.

I began to work with a therapist and I discovered some wonderful self-help books. I went to conferences and lectures about growth and self-care. It was a wonderful time of self-discovery and exponential growth. I began to experience true peace in my soul for the first time since I was a little girl.

At that time, I was introduced to the concept of a gratitude journal. In *Simple Abundance*, Sarah Ban Brathnach teaches the benefits of keeping a daily gratitude journal. I began a daily practice of gratitude.

My gratitude journal literally saved my life. As I learned to be grateful in life, I learned that I could take care of myself, that there were resources from the world that would support my journey, and that I have much to be grateful for.

As I turned that gratitude into a habit, it became easier to focus on the beauty of life and the joy that comes from gratitude.

Sometimes learning to be grateful can be difficult if we are in a difficult place. Trying to be grateful when so much feels wrong can seem like an impossible task. There are a few things that will help you to be able to move toward conscious gratitude. It begins by realizing that you do not have to have huge things to be grateful for.

When I first started my gratitude practice, I couldn't find anything to be grateful for, so I began to just say I was grateful for something. The things seemed silly at the time. I couldn't find deep gratitude, so I would be grateful that I could go to bed.

Then I learned to expand it to "I am grateful to sleep in a comfortable bed." Next I became grateful for sheets on the bed, for the farmers who grew the cotton for my comfy sheets, for the store clerk who sold me the sheets, and on and on.

Gratitude truly is a muscle that needs to be developed. The more you use it, the more grateful you become.

Begin by developing the following ten habits in your daily life:

1. Slow down. Breathe. Take three deep breaths to slow down your thinking and your bodily reactions.

2. Take a few moments to become conscious of your surroundings and become present to your situation. Allow the warm and peaceful feeling of stillness to permeate your body.

3. Embrace all the good around you. Gratitude can be for your first cup of coffee in the morning, for living in a beautiful location, for having your needs met, for sunshine . . . and more.

4. Write down at least six things you are grateful for every night in your gratitude journal. Before long, it will not be possible to keep it to just six. The more you are grateful, the more you have to be grateful for.

5. On a daily basis, take a few minutes to offer gratitude. Simply close your eyes and offer thanks to those around you. This awareness is the beginning of creating an "attitude of gratitude."

6. Remember what you were taught in kindergarten—simply saying "thank you" allows you to be more grateful. Every day we encounter people during our many activities. Say "thank you" to those you interact with—the hostess at the restaurant, the checkout person at the store, your significant other for being there, and maybe even your mom—for teaching you to say "thank you." The more you become aware of saying "thank you," the less you will focus on the negative around you.

7. During your gratitude journaling time, you may recall people for whom you are thankful or an act of kindness that impacted you. When that thought comes to mind, take a quick moment to make a phone call, send a text, or, my favorite: send a short handwritten note.

   I keep notes near my journal so that it's easy to pick up a card, write a few sentences, and mail it off. If you are not sure what to write, write a sentence or two sharing why you are grateful and add a quote on gratitude. In our busy culture, a handwritten note is a rarity. When you write one, you impact another person's life and may spark some gratitude in them.

8. Find or create your own gratitude. Each day choose a gratitude thought or quote, then write it out or post it as a background for your phone or computer. That way every time you get busy or forget to focus on what is good, you will have an instant reminder of gratitude.

9. Remember this powerful story on gratitude from the Jewish tradition:

   Once when times were tough, two men—both poor farmers—were walking down a country lane and met their Rabbi.

   "How is it for you?" the Rabbi asked the first man.

   "Lousy," he grumbled, bemoaning his lot and lack. "Terrible, hard, awful. Not worth getting out of bed for. Life is lousy."

   Now, God was eavesdropping on this conversation. "Lousy?" the Almighty thought. "You think your life is lousy now, you ungrateful lout? I'll show you what lousy is."

Then, the Rabbi turned to the second man. "And you, my friend?"

"Ah, Rabbi—life is good! God is so gracious, so generous. Each morning when I awaken, I'm so grateful for another day, for I know, rain or shine, it will unfold in wonder and blessings too bountiful to count. Life is so good."

God smiled as the second man's thanksgiving soared upward until it became one with the harmony of the heavenly hosts. Then the Almighty roared with delighted laughter. "Good? You think your life is good now? I'll show you what good is!"

10. Find or create your daily thought or prayer on gratitude. Each day, begin and end your day with this thought. This is one of my favorite gratitude prayers:

May you be well.

May you be happy.

May you be free from suffering.

May your life be full of gratitude.

As you allow gratitude to flow through your body the energy becomes joy.

FINDING YOUR WAY
7 Days of Gratitude Quotes (Example)

Day	I am Grateful
1	Gratitude changes the pangs of memory into a tranquil joy. — *Dietrich Bonhoeffer*
2	Feeling gratitude and not expressing it is like wrapping a present and not giving it. — *William Arthur Ward*
3	When you are grateful, fear disappears and abundance appears. — *Anthony Robbins*
4	We should certainly count our blessings, but we should also make our belssing count. — *Neal A. Maxwell*
5	Some people grumble that roses have thorns; I am grateful that thorns have roses. — *Alphonse Karr*
6	Acknowledging the good you already have in your life is the foundation for all abundance. — *Echkart Tolle*
7	This moment is your life. Remember it with gratitude. — *Jill Davis*

Download a printable worksheet at JillDavisCoaching.com/worksheets

FINDING YOUR WAY
7 Days of Gratitude Quotes

Day	I am Grateful
1	
2	
3	
4	
5	
6	
7	

Download a printable worksheet at JillDavisCoaching.com/worksheets

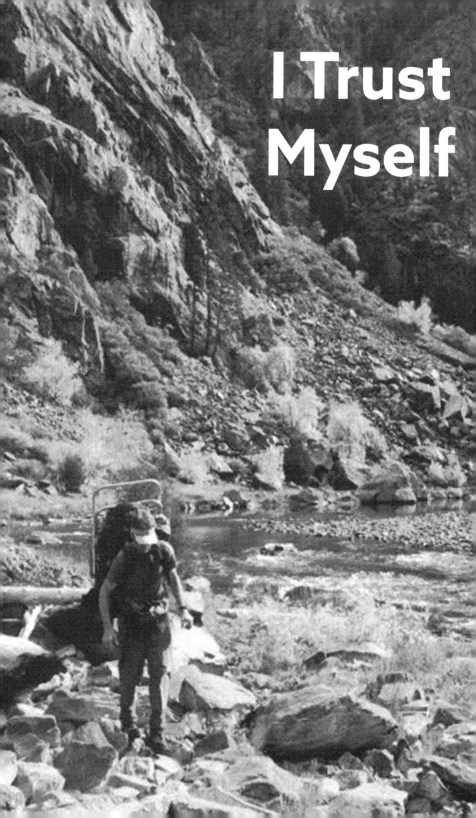

I Trust
Myself

CHAPTER 7

*I am comfortable looking
in the mirror and saying,
"I love you, I really love you."*

— *Louise Hay*

FOR MANY OF US who have spent years or decades overweight, positive affirmations can seem to be more frustrating than helpful. However, we must learn to offer unconditional love to our bodies and ourselves. Using positive affirmations and mirror work is one of the best ways to begin falling in love with your life.

Mirror work is a process in which you learn to see yourself in a more positive way. Louise Hay is often given credit for developing this concept. It is a simple and effective way to change your self-talk. When we change our self-talk, we see the world differently.

Our thoughts make us who we are. The way we talk to ourselves is the way we see ourselves. Often we will say things to ourselves that we would not say to our worst enemy.

To change our lives, we must change our self-talk and this can be done through mirror talk (also known as saying positive affirmations). Most often when we look in the mirror, we don't see ourselves; we simply see the reflection of ourselves. You might see how your hair looks or how you smile. What we don't usually do is look into our own eyes.

Mirror work is not just a way to think differently about yourself. The purpose is to really learn to value yourself—just as you are—and how you are created. It's a way to learn to love yourself so that you can return that love to the world, through both personal and business relationships. Because when we fall in love with our life and ourselves, our world will change.

The first step in mirror talk is to look into the mirror and look into your own eyes. Don't look past them to the mirror or around them or at your face; look deep into your eyes. Begin to see yourself as your own best friend.

Before you begin your mirror work:

1. Imagine what you want.

2. Decide the emotion that you want to feel.

3. Create your outcome.

4. Write it down.

5. Say it to yourself in the mirror daily.

6. Track your progress.

Mirror work is about using positive words, thoughts, and affirmations to recreate our world. Positive affirmations are not just a "hippy" idea or a salesperson's intention to try to make more money. New brain-science research shows that using the concept of positive words actually helps to rewire our brains which is possible because of the neuroplasticity of our brains.

Positive affirmations are a great way to start your mirror talk. Positive affirmations should be spoken in first person, in present tense, and be positive.

Positive Example:

"I love and bless my body and the way I feel at _____ pounds."

Negative Example:

"I am going to lose 35 pounds of ugly fat."

Positive Example:

"Every way and every day I am better at achieving my goals."

Negative Example:

"I don't care if it kills me; I'm going to accomplish my goals."

Choose the areas of your life that you want to improve. Choose your own truth. If you don't love your body right now, modify your affirmation to say a truth, such as "I love how my body allows me to accomplish my goals," or "My body is the exact right one for me."

As you build your positive affirmations, consider all areas of your life: physical, emotional, mental, relationships, career, and financial.

When you first begin to practice mirror work, you may feel uncomfortable, silly, or even angry. That's okay. It's part of the process. You will begin to see the part of your life that is keeping you stuck in a place you don't want to be. Keep practicing. As you say your affirmations, they will continue to become more real for you and you will experience the reality of your words.

Each day in your mirror work, tell yourself all of the affirmations you have created. As you grow in comfort in this area, choose your top three affirmations. Write these three down on a card or paper that you can carry with you. Every time you catch a reflection of yourself in a mirror, say these three affirmations until they are part of your memory and life. Repeat with the next three most relevant affirmations for you. As you do this over and over, these thoughts will become a part of your subconscious as well as your conscious life.

At the beginning, you might want to write down your positive affirmations so that you remember exactly what you want to say to yourself. By repeating your affirmations over and over, your subconscious mind will release your negative thoughts and replace them with positive thoughts. You may be surprised how quickly these words become a reality for you.

I have listed 95 affirmations to get you thinking. You may use them as they are written, or feel free to rewrite them in your own words. Only use the ones that are the truth for you. Put them everywhere you can think of, but most importantly, be sure to attach them to the mirror where you see yourself in the morning and at night .

Now, take a couple of deep breaths and begin to say your positive affirmations out loud. Look deep into your own eyes and speak into your life. Be sure to smile at yourself. Continue to breathe and speak your positive words for a few minutes. Over time, increase your mirror talk to five or ten minutes at least once a day.

Your mirror work should begin and end with the basic statement, "I love you." Too often we tell others just how much we love them, but forget to tell ourselves. When you love yourself, you will begin to face the world from an inner place that is infused with love. Every time you see yourself in a mirror say the three most important words: "I love you."

Although positive affirmations and mirror talk can change the way we feel and act, it is important to remember that sometimes life is just hard. In those times, remember to breathe, and simply love yourself. Offer yourself love even when you are sad, lonely, or worried. Loving yourself allows you to create healing in the sore spaces.

95 *Affirmations*

1. I give myself permission to say no when I am asked to do something that I really don't want to do.

2. I speak up for myself. I choose to accept responsibility for my own actions.

3. I choose to rest and heal when my body is tired. I do this without the need for justification.

4. I see each day as an opportunity to grow and to learn.

5. My days are filled with joy and interesting activities.

6. I choose my activities carefully. I choose those that nurture my soul and bring me happiness.

7. I live at peace with others and myself.

8. I am patient with external circumstances.

9. I embrace the changes that come with growth and I embrace the changes that flow through all aspects of my life.

10. Peace and joy are my guiding principles.

11. I live in a healthy body and my actions reflect my health.

12. I allow myself to receive love and to give love away.

13. I have abundance in both time and finances to accomplish all that I am called to do.

14. I bring love to my life, everyday, in all of my actions.

15. I create the change I want for my life.

16. I embrace my personality style and share my gift with the world.

17. I accept myself for who I am. I consciously embrace my life without judgment or criticism.

18. I take personal responsibility for my choices and actions. My life is up to me and I create the life of my dreams.

19. I respect myself.

20. I am congruent in my words and actions.

21. I honor the wisdom of my soul and I listen to my intuition.

22. I can achieve any dream that my mind conceives.

23. I choose to focus on the positive. I live in my victory story.

24. I embrace the past, without judgment, and all that I have learned from it.

25. I look toward the future with hope and anticipation of the outcome.

26. I live in prosperity and abundance in all aspects of my life.

27. I open my heart and mind to receive all that is necessary for my success.

28. I truly love my life and embrace my success.

29. I meet every challenge with the awareness that it will take me to my ultimate success.

30. I am capable of creating the life I desire.

31. I am happy with me. This is the ultimate success.

32. I am worthy of success in all areas of my life.

33. I welcome abundance in every part of my life.

34. I let go of my resistance to wealth and abundance in finances.

35. My needs are fully provided for by life.

36. I do the daily activities that are needed to create the success I desire.

37. I do not allow my fears to interfere with the abundance of my life.

38. I embrace my emotions and consciously choose my responses.

39. I choose to forgive and to let go of my anger.

40. I choose a beautiful life filled with joy and peace.

41. I move through challenging circumstances with grace.

42. My life is filled with laughter and fun.

43. I complete activities that propel me to my best life.

44. I am creative in all that I do.

45. I provide hope and encouragement to those around me.

46. I take time daily to bring fun into my life.

47. I know activity brings success. I take the actions that I need to create the success I want.

48. I give freely to others, being aware of the abundance of life.

49. I am grateful in all things.

50. I can take care of myself. I make good decisions every day.

51. I courageously confront all challenges on my path.

52. I stand my ground when faced with conflict. I believe in the strength of my decisions.

53. I inspire those around me.

54. Today is an opportunity to improve my life and the lives of others.

55. I release the past and embrace the present moment.

56. Nothing has energy, except for the energy I give it.

57. I consciously choose my actions.

58. I act instead of reacting.

59. I accept change easily.

60. I live my life from my personal choices, not from the decisions or desires of others.

61. I am uniquely gifted for my situation in life.

62. I have the courage to create the life I want.

63. I am willing to make mistakes.

64. I live the life I want and I want the life I live.

65. I surround myself with people who want the best for me.

66. I easily release relationships that are toxic for me.

67. I see obstacles in my path as opportunities for success.

68. Every day I stretch the boundaries of my belief.

69. I consistently widen my comfort zone as I step out of my current comfort.

70. I give more than people expect and I do it with joy.

71. I only allow people I respect to speak into my life.

72. I am successful because I am serving my purpose, not my problem.

73. My bigger-than-life goal is backed by a bigger-than-life mindset.

74. I receive wealth in all areas of my life.

75. Miracles surround me.

76. Love and prosperity flow freely into my life.

77. I appreciate all that I have.

78. I prosper in all that I do.

79. I communicate with clarity, wisdom, and humor.

80. I am open to new avenues of income.

81. I am grateful for the miracles that happen to me daily.

82. I make decisions that others won't.

83. I take action where others don't.

84. I give and receive love in abundance.

85. I radiate love and joy into the world.

86. I live in joy and abundance.

87. I am surrounded by love.

88. I choose to feed my body with healthy foods.

89. I eat when I am hungry; I stop when I am full.

90. I release my desire to control the future.

91. I trust myself.

92. My life unfolds easily and effortlessly.

93. I approve of myself, just the way I am.

94. I always find a way to bring about what I desire.

95. My life is the very one I want.

Over time, you will find your own personal affirmations that will bring hope, love, and joy.

FINDING YOUR WAY
7 Affirmations to Change
How You See the World (Example)

Day	Affirmation
1	I choose my activities carefully. I choose those that nurture my soul and bring me happiness.
2	I allow myself to receive love and to give love away.
3	I accept myself for who I am. I consciously embrace my life without judgment or criticism.
4	I embrace my personality style and share my gift with the world.
5	I look toward the future with hope and anticipation of the outcome.
6	I am happy with me. This is the ultimate success.
7	I do the daily activities that are needed to create the success I desire.

Download a printable worksheet at JillDavisCoaching.com/worksheets

FINDING YOUR WAY
7 Affirmations to Change
How You See the World

Day	Affirmation
1	
2	
3	
4	
5	
6	
7	

Download a printable worksheet at JillDavisCoaching.com/worksheets

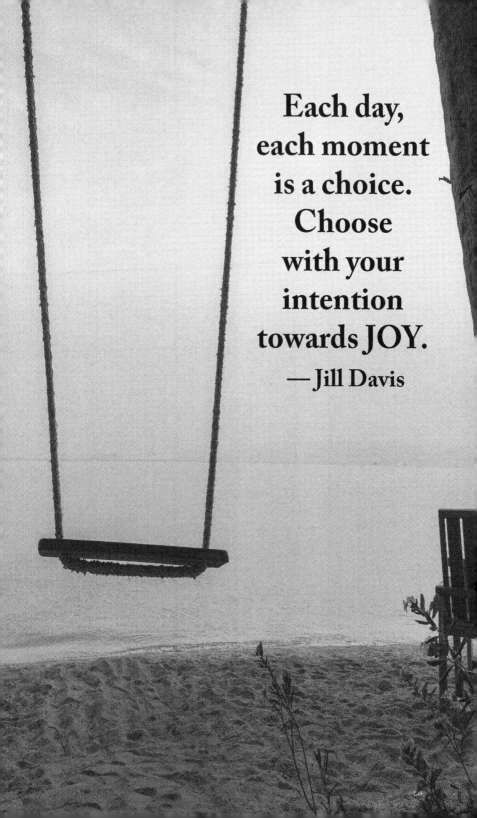

Each day,
each moment
is a choice.
Choose
with your
intention
towards JOY.
— Jill Davis

CHAPTER 8

*At times the world may seem an
unfriendly and sinister place, but believe
that there is much more good in it than
bad. All you have to do is look hard
enough and what might seem to be a
series of unfortunate events may in fact be
the first steps of a journey.*

— *Lemony Snicket*

DIETING IS HOW I began this journey. A series of unfortunate events. Diets don't work. We all know it. Yet we all do it. A Google search on weight loss delivered over 99 million results. Some of my favorite titles:

- 16 Ways to Lose Weight Fast
- 15 Teeny Tiny Ways to Lose Weight Faster
- How to Lose Belly Fat in 4 Days
- Lose 35 Pounds Without Working Out

- How to Lose 20 Pounds in 20 Days Without Changing Anything
- 40 Fast and Easy Tips to Losing Weight
- 10 Painless Ways to Lose Weight
- Weight Loss Shortcuts for Men
- How to Lose Weight Without Trying
- *And My Favorite:* How to Help your Dog Lose Weight

I have to admit, as I read through the titles, it was a bit tempting to go in and read the articles!

I still remember looking for that magic weight-loss pill. I am fascinated how the diet industry can keep saying the same thing over and over, and yet they generate over $60 billion a year in revenue.[10] Each one claims something different is their secret sauce, and despite decades of results falling short of their promises, the industry never misses a beat.

We continue to diet and diet. Each time it gets a little harder, but we are eternal optimists. We truly believe somehow this one will be the one we get right. In fact, the average American woman will spend more than 17 years of her lifetime on a diet.[11] I am certain that I skewed those averages. I dieted for way more than 17 years.

So we know diets don't work and yet we still keep dieting. Some people don't care; they just want to get to the good stuff or believe the delusion of "How to Lose 30 Pounds in 30 Minutes While Eating All the Ice Cream You Can Hold."

Each time you start a new diet, you probably think: "This time I'm really going to do it. I'm going to be good and not eat anything that is not on the list. I'm going to work out every day. This time is different."

Diets just don't work. Each year approximately 45 million people go on a diet and only five percent actually maintain significant weight loss. It's time to get off the roller coaster of weight loss and really start understanding that a restrictive diet won't create a healthy natural weight. Being healthy comes from learning to listen to your body and accepting who and how you are.

If diets worked, wouldn't they stop writing about it by now? We know they don't work, but why not? If you reduce your calories, shouldn't you lose weight?

The typical concept of weight loss is that reducing the caloric intake and increase the caloric output is the only effective way to lose weight. But it doesn't work. There are many reasons for this.

The Minnesota Experiment

One of the reasons is exhibited through a research program done just after WWII. It was called the Minnesota Experiment[12] and was conducted to understand the minimum amount of calories needed to sustain a human body beyond starvation.

Dr. Ancel Keys used conscientious objectors who were healthy and volunteered for the experiment. He reduced their calories from 3,200 a day to just 1,570 a day for a period of six months. These men, who started the experiment at a healthy weight, lost an average of 25 percent of their body weight.

When it was over, they went through a rehabilitation stage where they increased their calorie intake up to 4,000 a day until they had regained their weight. This rehabilitation stage lasted approximately 3 months.

The unexpected result of the experiment was the psychological impact of the dieting. The majority of the men said they spent much of their lives after this time thinking about food, wanting food, and eating even if they weren't hungry. Some of them would secretly consume as much as 11,000 calories in a day immediately after the rehabilitation period.

When I first read this study, I was very aware that my average diet had a calorie intake of anywhere from 700 calories to 1,200 calories, nowhere close to the 1,570 "starvation diet" Dr. Keys had created. Through the study, Keys realized that the men had been put into a starvation brain function, prompting the men's bodies to slow down their metabolism so as to retain fat. They became irritable, delusional, food-obsessed, and exhausted. That sounds exactly like me on a diet!

The Diet Brain

The starvation effect is very strong. When we diet, our brains go into survival mode. Our brains believe that we are literally starving (not our daily hunger) and our body becomes more efficient at storing fat. Our bodies and our brains cannot exist long-term without craving food and eventually binging on it to stop the hungry feeling.

And this is how the yo-yo dieting begins:

- We start a restrictive calorie or food diet.
- We stay on the diet for a few weeks, months, or even longer.
- We lose some weight, but we lose more lean muscle than fat as our bodies store the fat due to the famine we have put our bodies into.
- Our survival brains take over.
- We eat.
- We eat.
- WE EAT.
- And we finally stop feeling hungry.
- We get angry at ourselves for eating.
- And we go back into starvation and start the next "latest and greatest" diet.

Our bodies work just the way they were designed; during starvation, we store body fat to keep us alive. Only our survival brains don't know that we are living in a world of an abundance of food and that we are forcing ourselves into starvation. Our bodies start to hold on to fat so as to survive not just the past famine or diet but to survive the one it knows is coming.[13]

Every time we diet, we go back into this roller coaster, weight cycling pattern. Each time you listen to your body, avoid starvation, pay attention to your body fuel gauge, and love yourself, you are taking one step closer to the healthy body that you want.

It doesn't matter if this is the 100th time or more that you've told yourself, "Today I am going to stop dieting." Now is the time. No more dieting and no more hating on yourself. Keep trusting who you are and that your body knows best.

As you begin this Food Journey and stop fighting your weight and yourself, I know that you will begin to find your way. I am excited for this amazing life journey you are on. I celebrate you. Breathe. Be present. Be grateful.

Be BRAVE.
Be BEAUTIFUL.
Be YOU.

CONCLUSION

*M*Y FINAL WEIGHT IS around 135 to 140 pounds. My total weight loss is at least 120 pounds but most likely closer to 130 pounds. I still have days where I would rather eat sugar than face what's in front of me. I have developed tools that help to move me past that place and into self-acceptance, love, and peace—tools that help me to have courage, clarity, and confidence to take on life on life's terms.

These are basic concepts that can be experienced and learned.

- Trust yourself.
- Learn your hunger and fullness signals.
- Practice gratitude.
- Learn to love yourself.
- Become active.
- Understand how you are wired.
- Listen to your intuition.
- Fall in love with life.

I used to think if I could just be skinny, everything would be fine. Then I thought if I could just be fit, everything would be fine. Now I know everything is not always fine, but I can always find joy in the process. I found the tools that I could use, and created the ones that I couldn't find.

I learned to love to move my body in many ways. I adventured back into the great outdoors. I moved into true health and discovered my true authentic body, which is the home in which my authentic soul resides.

The most important part of my weight release is the reclaiming of my life. I chose to figure out what was inside me that kept me fat—the emotions that drove me to try to fill up with overeating—and to learn to stop eating my pain and emptiness. I continue to discover more and more about myself every day.

I learned that it is not what size I wear. It doesn't matter if I am a size six or a size ten or a size twenty-four. It simply matters that I embrace today, find the joy where I can, and truly fall in love with my life. It changed everything.

You can do it, too. I believe in you. Whatever you are fighting with food, you will win the battle. As you stop fighting your weight, you will find your way. You are **Brave**. You are **Beautiful**. You are **You**!

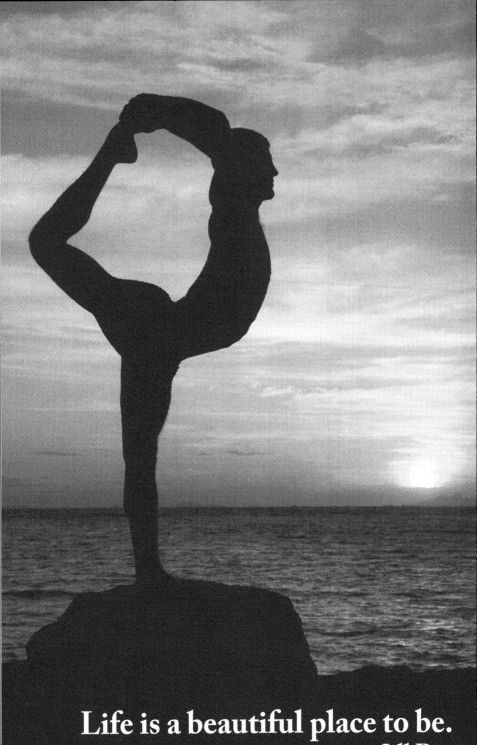

Life is a beautiful place to be.
—Jill Davis

GRATITUDE

Gratitude has been part of my life for so long and yet it always brings me to tears when I think of all the amazing people who have allowed me to be part of their world as they have become part of my world.

I am grateful for:

Jamie Fletcher, for being my love, my joy, my partner. This is an exciting life. I can't wait to share it with you. Thank you for teaching me that we never know if we will have tomorrow so let's celebrate the joy of today!

Emily Chase Smith, who believed in me when I couldn't believe in myself. I can't imagine doing life without your friendship.

James Woosley, who has the patience of a saint. You held my hand and helped me see that with the right partner a book was really possible. I never wanted to write this book, but I knew I wanted to get the message out to more people. You made that happen.

Megan Miks, my friend from forever who stepped in and changed a stock photo idea into a reality. I am beyond grateful for the many years of friendship and a rocking photo as well.

Valeria Spencer and Cathy Karmondy, for holding my hand and my heart through this crazy transformation and keeping all my private stories private. The years have only made us better.

Rhonda Koehn, who taught me how to have great hair while teaching me that love and friendship comes in many varied and unexpected forms. Thank you for seeing me through all these years.

Kent Julian, who showed up in my life right when I needed a mentor…and then became a dear friend.

Andrea Rose, because you are the tech goddess and you allowed me to look fabulous online even when I didn't feel fabulous offline.

All of the women who trusted me to coach them through the process of finding their way and then allowing me to put their experiences into practice through this book.

All my sisters of the heart: Carolyn Selvig, Anna Compton, Anne Marlow, Jessica Arent, Maggie Barentine, Barbara Cardona, Carla Boomgarden, LaRa Fryer, Diana Bader, Tiffany Montavon, Emily Montavon, Kim Miller, Juliet Pattullo, Laurie Wilson, Jacquie Fedo, Lori Niell, Jeanette Bogart, Jen McDonough, Robin Stephenson, Martha Chinnock, Michelle Johnson, Dorothy Sander, Suzanne Caplan, Joanne Miller, Ashley Logsdon, Stephanie Johnson, Susan Mcbroom, and Ashley Eaton. Each of you walked with me on this journey in your own brave, beautiful way.

Scheila Watson, Jude Blitz, and Sharon Mauldin for providing the therapy and coaching I needed to move through my trauma places

My beautiful family of origin that gave me many gifts, including some of them wrapped in oddly shaped packages. Each gift is received with joy.

Kim Novitske, for showing up at the right time with the right skill set to make the end of this writing process so much easier.

Rich Herrmann, for showing up in my life and instantly becoming my friend, my confidant, my support. I was waiting for you.

Daphne DePorres, for listening to me say the TEDx talk over and over and over and over and over and over and.... I couldn't have done this without you.

Kent Montavon, for teaching me so many life lessons in so many interesting ways. Sunrises, sunsets, coffee, and birds on the wing—I will never forget you.

Larry Sutton, Jamie Slingerland, Pierce Marrs, Nick Pavlidis, Jay Parks, Xander Page, Scott Werner, Jeff McManus, Bob Kittridge, Roger Whitney, Steve Bonham, Brett Davidson, Charles Jones, Jake Lohwater, and Jeremy Myers. Each of you taught me that there really are good men out there.

To all my mentors that I never met from whom I absorbed every possible bit of knowledge from your writings and podcasts.

For each of you who touched my life along the way and allowed me to be a part of your life... there are just too many to list. If you have read to this point, please know you are the one for whom I am grateful.

I am beyond grateful for this life.
It is a beautiful place to be.

MINI DISC PROFILE

How are You Wired?

Take the Mini DISC profile to gain a basic understanding of your personality. You can visit JillDavisCoaching.com/store to purchase an in depth DISC assessment.

For each question, circle the item that most fits who you are. If you are not sure, remember a time that you felt really comfortable in being you and answer from that place. If two answers feel appropriate, pick based on your initial instinct.

1) When faced with a difficult task, I need to:	A	Create a motivational environment
	B	Take charge of the environment
	C	Create a cooperative environment
	D	Follow key directives and best practices

2) When walking into a conference room:	A	I'll be checking to see if anyone needs help
	B	I tend to be in charge so I am there early
	C	I have my color-coded pens laid out for notes and am ready to start on time
	D	I will find a spot with my friends

3) The most difficult part of a team meeting is when:	A	It goes on too long and gets boring
	B	People don't listen to my advice
	C	When we don't follow the agenda
	D	When I don't know the people well

4) When telling a joke:	A	I have some great one-liners and a dry sense of humor
	B	I can make any story funny, but sometimes it takes too long to tell it
	C	Sometimes people think I am serious when I am really joking
	D	I like a good joke but not if it hurts someone's feelings

5) The decision-making process is:	A	Something I hope someone else will handle
	B	Easy because I get excited about new adventures
	C	Long and slow because I need time to study all the facts before I decide
	D	Easy for me because I'm usually right

6) When I face a problem in a group environment:	A	I like to make sure things get done quickly
	B	I like to make sure everything gets done in an orderly manner
	C	I like to make sure everyone is having fun during the process
	D	I like to make sure everyone is comfortable

7) When making friends:	A	I have lots of friends because I'm easygoing and a good listener
	B	I make friends easily; people are drawn to me
	C	I like having a few close friends and am careful to choose loyal ones
	D	I like to be the leader and people like to follow me

8) I can get frustrated when:	A	I'm put in an unfamiliar setting
	B	People don't get along
	C	I am not acknowledged for the work I do
	D	People don't like me

9) I love when:	A	I get to go out for a night with my friends
	B	My family is together for game night
	C	I tackle a task and finish it quickly
	D	My to-do list is completed

10) I don't like:	A	Losing control
	B	Feeling less than
	C	Losing popularity
	D	Being wrong

Transfer your answers from the questions onto the key below. For example, if you answered question 1 with answer C, then the result is **S**. Write that in the Result column. Then count the number of **D**s, **I**s, **S**s, and **C**s in the totals section at the bottom. The highest number will give you a basic indication of your primary DISC personality trait.

Question	Key				Result
1	A	B	C	D	
	I	D	S	C	
2	A	B	C	D	
	S	D	C	I	
3	A	B	C	D	
	I	D	C	S	
4	A	B	C	D	
	C	I	D	S	
5	A	B	C	D	
	S	I	C	D	
6	A	B	C	D	
	D	C	I	S	
7	A	B	C	D	
	S	I	C	D	
8	A	B	C	D	
	C	S	D	I	
9	A	B	C	D	
	I	S	D	C	
10	A	B	C	D	
	D	S	I	C	

TOTAL	D	I	S	C

Download a printable worksheet at JillDavisCoaching.com/worksheets

RECOMMENDED READING

Steering by Starlight
by Martha Beck

Finding Your Own North Star
by Martha Beck

Challenge Accepted!:
A Simple Strategy for Living Life on Purpose
by James Woosley

Simple Abundance
by Sarah Ban Breathnach

What to Say When You Talk to Yourself
by Dr. Shad Helmstetter

The Go-Giver
by Bob Burg and John David Mann

The Joy Diet
by Martha Beck

If I'm So Smart Why Cant I Lose Weight
by Brooke Castillo

You Can Heal Your Life
by Louise Hay

Women, Food, and God
by Geneen Roth

A Course in Weight Loss
by Marianne Williams

The Body Never Lies
by Anne Miller

150 Pounds Gone Forever
by Diane Carbonell

703:
How I Lost More Than Quarter Ton and Gained a Life
by Nancy Makin

The Body Keeps the Score:
Brain, Mind, and Body in the Healing of Trauma
by Bessel van der Kolk, MD

Don't Let Anything Dull Your Sparkle:
How to Break Free of Negativity and Drama
by Doreen Virtue

Intuitive Eating
by Evelyn Tribole and Elyse Resch

Diana, Herself:
An Allegory of Awakening
(The Bewilderment Chronicles Book 1)
by Martha Beck

The Language of the Body
by Dr. Alexander Lowen M.D.

Constant Craving:
What Your Food Cravings Mean and How to Overcome Them
by Doreen Virtue

Big Magic:
Creative Living Beyond Fear
by Elizabeth Gilbert

The Big Leap:
Conquer Your Hidden Fear and Take Life to the Next Level
by Gay Hendricks, PhD

In an Unspoken Voice:
How the Body Releases Trauma and Restores Goodness
by Peter A. Levine, PhD

Losing Your Pounds of Pain
by Doreen Virtue

She Spoke Like Poetry
by Gracie Packard

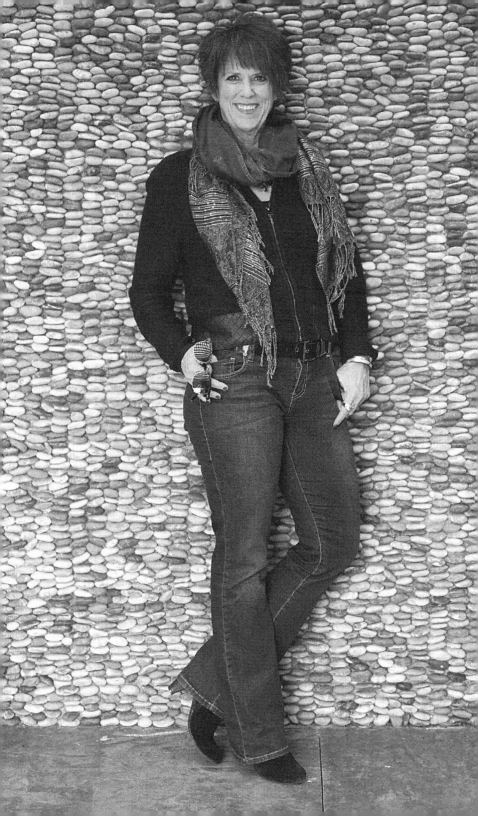

ABOUT THE AUTHOR

Jill Davis spent the majority of her adult life morbidly obese. She lost 135 pounds and along the way regained her identity. Through her own journey, research, and working with thousands of women in transition, Jill discovered that the move from body shaming to body acceptance is only possible when we shed the belief that we are intrinsically good or bad based on the foods we eat and instead trust our bodies to tell us what they need. When we embrace ourselves, we can explore the possibilities of who we can become and discover the best in ourselves.

Through workshops, keynote speaking, and one-on-one coaching, Jill helps others to quit fighting their weight and start finding their way. Jill is honored to have been invited to share her presentation "You Are Not Your Diet Brain" at TEDx.

Jill lives in the beautiful Rocky Mountains where she dotes on her granddaughter Maggie and loves on her four children, her partner, and the world.

Connect

Website:
JillDavisCoaching.com

Facebook:
Facebook.com/JillDavisCoaching

Twitter:
@AskJillDavis

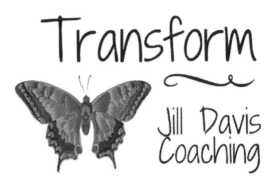

Transform

Jill Davis Coaching

Dear Reader:

This may be the end of the book, but it is not the end of your journey...

My greatest desire in life is to be a guide for you on your journey.

Are you tired of dieting and fighting the battle? You know now that diets don't work and anything that creates rules is a "diet." Join me as you continue to find your way and stop fighting your weight.

Learn more at JillDavisCoaching.com/finding-your-way and find the program that works best for you.

Jill

One-on-one Coaching
Private coaching tailored to your personal journey

Includes:

Access to private Facebook Page

Tips and advice

Support from the community

Topics and Support from Jill

Special Discounts on other products

Group Coaching
Group Coaching Calls

Sessions forming regularly

Access to private Facebook Page

Great tips and advice

Support from the community

Topics and Support from Jill

Special Discounts on other products

Private Support Group

Access to private Facebook Page

Great tips and advice

Support from the community

Topics and Support from Jill

Special Discounts on other coaching products

Speaking

And I would love to come speak to you and your group.

I love being around those people who want to be on this journey.

REFERENCES

1   *Food, mood and health: a neurobiologic outlook*
    Brazilian Journal of Medical and Biological Research (1998)
    31 (12):1517-1527
    DOI: 10.1590/S0100-879X1998001200002
    Chandan Prasad
    Section of Endocrinology & Metabolism, Department of
    Medicine, LSU Medical Center, New Orleans, LA, USA, 1998.

2   *Physiology & Behavior*
    Volume 38, Issue 4, October 1986, Pages 459–464.
    Dr. Kelly D. Brownell, Department of Psychiatry, University of
    Pennsylvania, 133 South 36th Street, Philadelphia, PA 19104.
    Copyright © 1986 Published by Elsevier Inc.

3   Davis CM. Self selection of diet by newly weaned infants: an
    experimental study. Am J Dis Child 1928;36(4):651-79 [reprinted
    as a Nutrition Classics article in Nutr Rev 1986;44:114-6].

4   *The Common Sense Book of Baby and Child Care* (page 218)
    Dr. Benjamin Spock
    New York: Duell, Sloan and Pearce; 1946

5   *Physiology & Behavior*
    Volume 38, Issue 4, October 1986, Pages 459–464.
    Dr. Kelly D. Brownell, Department of Psychiatry, University of
    Pennsylvania, 133 South 36th Street, Philadelphia, PA 19104.
    Copyright © 1986 Published by Elsevier Inc.

6   http://iffgd.org/symptoms-causes/abdominal-noises.html

7   http://www.ncbi.nlm.nih.go/pubmed/8697046

8   https://www.nationaleatingdisorders.org/what-body-image

9   *Forbes* – March 2015
     http://www.forbes.com/sites/vanessaloder/2015/03/18/how-
     to-rewire-your-brain-for-happiness/#69a78f4a3cb3

10   http://www.medicaldaily.com/average-woman-spends-17-
     years-her-life-diets-242601

11   http://www.marketdataenterprises.com/wp-content/
     uploads/2014/01/Diet-Market-2014-Status-Report.pdf
     • Marketdata, a market research firm that has tracked diet
       products and programs since 1989 releases its findings in its
       biennial study: "The U.S. Weight Loss & Diet Control Market."
       which in its 2007 study estimates the size of the U.S. weight
       loss market at $55 billion. It is now estimated to have
       reached over $60 Billion.

12   Minnesota Experiment
     • Minnesota project: http://jn.nutrition.org/
       content/135/6/1347.full
     • Kalm, L.M. & R.D. Semba (June 1, 2005) "They starved so
       that others be better fed: remembering Ancel Keys and
       the Minnesota experiment." The Journal of Nutrition 135(6):
       1347-1352.
     • Tucker, T. (2006). *The Great Starvation Experiment: The
       Heroic Men Who Starved So That Millions Could Live*. Simon
       & Schuster, Inc., New York.
     • Keys, A., Brozek, J., Henschel, A., Mickelsen, O. & Taylor, H.L.
       (1950) *The Biology of Human Starvation, Vols. I-II*. University
       of Minnesota Press, Minneapolis, MN.
     • "Men Starve in Minnesota" (July 30, 1945). Life 19(5): 43-46.

13   Development and psychometric evaluation of a measure of
     intuitive eating.
     Tylka, Tracy L.
     Journal of Counseling Psychology, Vol 53(2), Apr 2006, 226-
     240.
     http://dx.doi.org/10.1037/0022-0167.53.2.226

Learn More at

JILLDAVISCOACHING.COM

Made in the USA
Middletown, DE
29 October 2016